Epilepsy

616.853 B851eh
Buchanan, Neil.
 Epilepsy

To Jolyon:- to a place in the sun

Epilepsy
A Handbook

Neil Buchanan

Department of Paediatrics and the Epilepsy Unit
Westmead Hospital
Sydney 2145
Australia

W.B. SAUNDERS COMPANY LTD
London   Philadelphia   Toronto   Sydney   Tokyo

W. B. Saunders Company Ltd 24–28 Oval Road
London NW1 7DX

The Curtis Center
Independence Square West
Philadelphia, PA 19106–3399, USA

Harcourt Brace & Company
55 Horner Avenue
Toronto, Ontario M8Z 4X6, Canada

Harcourt Brace & Company, Australia
30–52 Smidmore Street
Marrickville, NSW 2204, Australia

Harcourt Brace & Company, Japan Inc
Ichibancho Central Building, 22–1 Ichibancho
Chiyoda-ku, Tokyo 102, Japan

© 1995 W. B. Saunders Company Ltd

Second printing 1995

This book is printed on acid free paper

All rights reserved. No part of this publication may be reproduced, stored in a retrieval system or transmitted, in any form or by any means, electronic, mechanical, photocopying or otherwise, without the prior permission of W. B. Saunders Company Ltd, 24–28 Oval Road, London NW1 7DX, England

A catalogue record for this book is available from the British Library

ISBN 0–7020–2014–1

Typeset by J&L Composition Ltd, Filey, North Yorkshire
Printed in Great Britain by George Over Ltd, Rugby

KENT FREE LIBRARY

Contents

Abbreviations		vii
Preface		ix
1	The classification of seizures and epilepsy	1
2	The aetiology, epidemiology and prognosis of epilepsy	13
3	Making the diagnosis	18
4	Medical management	28
5	Surgical management	56
6	Epilepsy in particular situations: the neonatal period, childhood, the elderly, pregnancy, the disabled and photosensitivity	59
7	Pseudo-epileptic seizures	68
8	Psychosocial issues	72
9	Epilepsy and lifestyle	81
10	Information for patients	86
References		89
Appendices		
(1) Drugs in development		94
(2) Epilepsy centres		95
(3) Epilepsy associations		98
(4) Further reading		102
Index		103

Abbreviations

Seizures/epilepsy

BFE	=	Benign focal epilepsy of childhood
CPS	=	Complex partial seizure
FC	=	Febrile convulsion
GTCS	=	Generalized tonic–clonic seizure
JME	=	Juvenile myoclonic epilepsy
LGD	=	Lennox–Gastaut syndrome
PES	=	Pseudo-epileptic seizure
PS	=	Partial seizure
SPS	=	Simple partial seizure

Investigations

CT	=	Computed tomography
EEG	=	Electroencephalography
MRI	=	Magnetic resonance imaging
PET	=	Positron emission tomography
SPECT	=	Single photon emission computed tomography
VEEG	=	Video-EEG telemetry

Routes of drug administration

IM	=	intramuscular
IV	=	intravenous

PO = oral
PR = rectal

■ Anti-epileptic drugs (AEDs)

Acetazolamide	AZM	Lorazepam	LZP
Carbamazepine	CBZ	Nitrazepam	NZP
Clobazam	CLB	Oxcarbazepine	OCBZ
Clonazepam	CZP	Phenobarbitone	PB
Diazepam	DZP	Phenytoin	PHT
Ethosuximide	ESM	Primidone	PRM
Felbamate	FBM	Sodium valproate	VPA
Gabapentin	GBP	Tiagabine	TGB
Lamotrigine	LTG	Topiramate	TPM
		Vigabatrin	VGB

Preface

Epilepsy is a relatively common condition. About 60–70% of people with epilepsy will be well controlled with anti-epileptic drugs (AEDs) and a good proportion of them will later go into remission and come off medication. Some 30% of people develop chronic epilepsy with seizures which are difficult to control, attend hospitals frequently and in the main are those with epilepsy whom medical students, residents and registrars are acquainted with. From a medical view point, it is this chronic group who occupy most attention. They are, however, not a reflection of epilepsy in the general community. Because of the nature of seizures including their physical manifestations, unpredictability and the psychological problems associated with chronic epilepsy, psychosocial problems are not uncommon. Further, people with epilepsy may feel stigmatized. While this is probably more often perceived than real, it may present an important facet of management for the practitioner.

There are also a number of important lifestyle issues which pertain to people with epilepsy. Obtaining a driving licence, career choices, pregnancy, late nights and alcohol ingestion are examples of topics upon which practitioners will be asked for advice. None of these issues is black and white, often requiring a common-sense approach. The management (rather than "treatment") of epilepsy requires the recognition that whilst patients with epilepsy go to doctors for assistance, their condition has particular social implications. Management must include attention to these social factors and not concentrate solely on the taking of medication, however important this is.

Most books on epilepsy appear somewhat daunting, thus the need for a relatively simple handbook providing a brief overview of the subject. It is hoped that this will be of use to health-care professionals, medical students and those who care for people with epilepsy.

By virtue of the intentional brevity of this book, it will not be possible to discuss issues in detail. The intent is to provide a brief, factual overview of an important condition with which all practitioners will be confronted from time to time. There have been considerable advances in epileptology over the past decade with new investigational techniques, a burgeoning of new drugs and considerable progress with surgical treatment. The outlook for people with epilepsy is a deal better than it has been, which will be reflected in this handbook!

The book is intended to be an easy read and is expressly written in plain language: not a textbook, but a handbook. The author is indebted to Dr. Mark Richardson, Dr. Rod McKenzie and Dr. Paddy Grattan-Smith for comments on the manuscript and to Mrs. Eve Otmar for its recurrent typing.

Neil Buchanan

1 The classification of seizures and epilepsy

Epilepsy is manifested by recurrent seizures with a seizure being an intermittent, stereotyped disturbance. The disturbance may be of consciousness, motor function, behaviour, perception, sensation and emotion or a combination of any of these.

Seizures may vary from person to person, but are individually stereotyped. Seizures are classified according to their onset: partial or generalized (**Table 1**)[1]. Partial seizures are subdivided according to consciousness during the episode: retained in simple partial seizures (SPS) and impaired to a varying extent in complex partial seizures (CPS). An aura is a simple partial seizure. Any partial seizure has the potential to secondarily generalize to a tonic–clonic seizure (GTCS).

While there are a number of seizure types, there are numerous forms of epilepsy syndromes which are defined by age of onset, seizure types, electroencephalogram (EEG) changes and associated clinical features.

The main value of a syndromic classification is that by grouping like patients and following them up, it is

Partial seizures

Simple (consciousness retained)
  With motor symptoms
  With sensory symptoms
  With autonomic symptoms
  With psychic manifestations

Complex (consciousness impaired)
  With impairment of consciousness only
  With automatisms
  Partial seizures which secondarily generalize

Generalized seizures

  Absence seizures – typical and atypical
  Myoclonic seizures
  Clonic seizures
  Tonic seizures
  Tonic–clonic seizures
  Atomic seizures

Table 1 The classification of seizures. Modified from the Commission on Classification and Terminology of the International League Against Epilepsy (ILAE)[1]

1. Localization – related (focal, local, partial) epilepsies and syndromes
   1.1 Idiopathic (with age-related onset)
       benign childhood epilepsy with centrotemporal spike
       childhood epilepsy with occipital paroxysms
       primary reading epilepsy
   1.2 Symptomatic
       chronic progressive epilepsia partialis continua of childhood (Kojewnikow's syndrome)
       syndromes characterized by seizures with specific modes of presentation
   1.3 Cryptogenic (presumed symptomatic but aetiology unknown)
2. Generalized epilepsies and syndromes
   2.1 Idiopathic (with age-related onset, listed in order of age)

benign neonatal familial convulsions
benign neonatal convulsions
benign myoclonic epilepsy in infancy
childhood absence epilepsy
juvenile absence epilepsy
juvenile myoclonic epilepsy
epilepsy with grand mal (generalized tonic–clonic seizures) on awakening
other generalized idiopathic epilepsies not defined above
epilepsies with seizures precipitated by specific modes of activation (reflex and reading epilepsies)
2.2 Cryptogenic or symptomatic (in order of age)
West syndrome
Lennox–Gastaut syndrome
epilepsy with myoclonic–astatic seizures
epilepsy with myoclonic absences
2.3 Symptomatic
2.3.1 Non-specific aetiology
early myoclonic encephalopathy
early infantile epileptic encephalopathy with suppression burst
other symptomatic generalized epilepsies not defined above
2.3.2 Specific syndromes/aetiologies
cerebral malformations
inborn errors of metabolism including pyridoxine dependency and disorders frequently presenting as progressive myoclonic epilepsy
3. Epilepsies and syndromes undetermined, whether focal or generalized
3.1 With both generalized and focal seizures
neonatal seizures
severe myoclonic epilepsy in infancy
epilepsy with continuous spike waves during slow-wave sleep

> acquired epileptic aphasia (Landau–Kleffner syndrome)
> other undetermined epilepsies not defined above
> 3.2 Without unequivocal generalized or focal features

Table 2 The ILAE classification of epilepsy[2]

Neonatal
Benign familial neonatal seizures
Benign neonatal seizures
Pyridoxine dependency
Myoclonic epilepsy
 benign
 severe

Infancy
West syndrome (infantile spasms)
Myoclonic epilepsy
 benign
 severe

Young children (1–5 years)
Febrile convulsions
Lennox–Gastaut syndrome

Older children (5–10 years)
Absence epilepsy
Benign partial epilepsy with centrotemporal spikes
Benign partial epilepsy with occipital spikes
Landau–Kleffner syndrome

Adolescence
Juvenile myoclonic epilepsy
Grand mal seizures on awakening
Absence epilepsy of adolescence

Table 3 The commoner epilepsy syndromes of epilepsy in childhood and adolescence

The classification of seizures and epilepsy

becoming possible to better define prognosis. It is also of some value in selecting appropriate treatment. The current International League Against Epilepsy (ILAE) classification of epilepsy, daunting though it is, is shown in **Table 2**, largely to demonstrate the complexity of the problem.[2] From a more practical, clinical point of view, the commoner epilepsy syndromes in childhood and adolescence can be looked at in an age-related fashion (**Table 3**). Some of these will be discussed in more detail.

■ Childhood epilepsy syndromes

▌ Benign familial neonatal seizures

A relatively uncommon condition of autosomal dominant inheritance occurring on the 2nd or 3rd day of life. Seizures are usually generalized and may occur many times a day, usually resolving in the first few months of life. Prognosis is excellent with a normal neurological outcome, although 1 in 7 of these infants may later develop epilepsy.[3]

▌ Benign neonatal seizures

Frequently called "5th day fits", this is an uncommon condition of clonic or subtle seizures (including apnoea) in healthy infants. Aetiology is uncertain, the outlook is excellent and epilepsy does not develop subsequently.

▌ Pyridoxine dependency[4]

A rare condition with seizures usually commencing on the first day of life. The episodes are usually generalized and do not respond to standard anti-epileptic drugs (AEDs). A therapeutic trial of pyridoxine (up to 100 mg IV) should be instituted as soon as the condition is suspected. The seizures will usually cease immediately. It should be remembered that apnoea can occur with IV pyridoxine administered in the neonatal period.

Myoclonic epilepsy in infancy

Benign: A rare condition with brief episodes of myoclonus in the first year of life in normal children with a family history of epilepsy. Sodium valproate is the AED of choice with the seizures being easily controlled. Some of these children may develop GTCS in adolescence.

Severe: A rare condition occurring in normal infants who develop myoclonic seizures, usually in the first few months of life. Development regresses and neurological signs may develop. Family clustering may occur with this condition which is often resistant to AEDs. The outlook for intellectual functioning is poor.

West syndrome (infantile spasms)

This syndrome consists of seizures, developmental delay and hypsarrhythmia on EEG. The seizures are myoclonic or tonic, leading to flexor or extensor spasms. The condition is relatively uncommon, occurring more often in boys and commencing between 3 and 12 months of age. If the child is able to sit, flexor spasms lead to the head and trunk going forwards (salaam attacks). If the child is not yet sitting, the seizures are often manifested by extensor spasms similar to a startle response.

In about 70% of cases, an aetiology can be defined: perinatal asphyxia, metabolic disorders, previous meningitis or cerebral malformations including tuberous sclerosis. The prognosis is worse in the "symptomatic" group than in the remaining 30% with no clear cause. Treatment remains difficult with frequent resistance to standard AEDs. Sodium valproate, clobazam, clonazepam and steroids are the most used agents. Vigabatrin offers new hope for the "symptomatic" group, especially with tuberous sclerosis. Spasms are quite often controlled, interestingly with the subsequent development of partial seizures requiring treatment in their own right.[5]

Lennox–Gastaut syndrome (LGS)

This condition occurs between 1 and 5 years of age, comprising seizures, a slow spike-and-wave EEG and moderate-to-severe intellectual retardation. The seizures include absences, jerking episodes (tonic and myoclonic seizures), atonic seizures or GTCS.

Many of the aetiological factors described for West syndrome may occur in LGS and indeed a proportion of patients with infantile spasms may progress to LGS. Treatment, as for West syndrome is difficult, although two of the new AEDs appear promising. Both lamotrigine[6,7] and felbamate[8,9] have been reported to be effective in LGS. Felbamate use has recently been associated with a number of cases of aplastic anaemia and severe hepatotoxicity. The future of this AED is uncertain. In view of the poor response to conventional AEDs, it may be that lamotrigine might become first-line therapy.

Febrile convulsions (FC)

In the classification of epilepsy and epilepsy syndromes, febrile convulsions (FC) are classified as situation-related seizures. As febrile convulsions do not go on to become epilepsy, it seems incongruous to include the topic in a book on epilepsy. This is done because

FC are the commonest cause of seizures in childhood, occurring in 3–4% of children. By definition, FC occur in neurodevelopmentally normal children between 6 months and 5 years of age in association with fever and in the absence of acute brain disease (e.g., encephalitis and meningitis) and can be divided into simple and complex FC.

Simple FC: These are brief (< 15 minutes), generalized and with no neurological sequelae. Recurrences occur with 37% having one subsequent FC, 30% two more FC and 17% at least three subsequent FC.[10] The most vulnerable period for recurrences is from 1 to 2 years of age.

Complex FC: These last > 15 minutes and are focal, perhaps associated with status epilepticus or with residual neurological signs (e.g. Todd's paresis).

A recent community-based study showed that 6 of 95 children with complex FC, as opposed to 3 of 287 with simple FC, subsequently developed epilepsy.[11] The latter figure of about 1 in 100 approximates the frequency of epilepsy in the general population. Prophylactic AED therapy is rarely required. When it is, a choice exists between maintenance therapy orally with phenobarbitone or sodium valproate, or intermittent therapy with rectal diazepam or oral diazepam.[12]

Prolonged FC may lead to the development of mesial temporal (hippocampal) sclerosis which may subsequently lead to the development of complex partial seizures (temporal lobe epilepsy). How frequently this occurs is uncertain.

■ Absence epilepsy

Contrary to common belief, absence epilepsy is uncommon, representing only 4–5% of childhood epilepsy. It is commoner in girls, usually beginning

The classification of seizures and epilepsy

between 3 and 10 years of age. Absence epilepsy is characterized by a sudden cessation of mental functioning during which the child is quite still with a vacant stare. The episodes last 5–15 seconds, ceasing as abruptly as they began although it may take a few more seconds for complete cerebral function to return. The presence of clonic movements or automatisms leads to the condition being called "complex typical absences", although this term is not universally used. The EEG shows a characteristic discharge of generalized, symmetrical spike and wave complexes at 3 Hz.

The seizures may be brief and subtle, may occur many times a day and patients may come to attention due to learning difficulties. Diagnostically, absences may be induced by hyperventilation for 2–3 minutes. Typical absence epilepsy usually responds well to treatment, with sodium valproate being the drug of choice. Ethosuximide is an alternative and lamotrigine seems to be of value in resistant patients. In about 50% of cases, GTCS will later develop. This makes the prognosis for complete remission less likely as does the onset of absences in late childhood or adolescence. Typical absence epilepsy usually remits in adolescence and never commences *de novo* in adult life.

Atypical absence epilepsy implies absence seizures not associated with a typical 3 Hz spike–wave pattern. The onset of atypical absences is less abrupt, they are often associated with other problems (e.g. LGS) and are less responsive to AEDs than typical absences.

Benign partial epilepsy with centrotemporal spikes[13]

This condition, also known as benign focal epilepsy (BFE), is common, representing 10–20% of childhood epilepsy. The onset is from 3 to 11 years of age with a peak from 5 to 8 years. It occurs more commonly in boys, with seizures consisting of paraesthesia involving the tongue, legs and cheek on one side or unilateral motor involvement of the face, lips, tongue, laryngeal and pharyngeal muscles leading to speech arrest, dysarthria and drooling with full retention of consciousness. About 20% of patients will have secondarily generalized tonic–clonic seizures. The parents are usually alerted by a gurgling sound, as if the child is choking. The episodes often occur in the early morning, with GTCS also arising from sleep. The frequency of seizures in BFE is often low, with about 25% having only one attack, half have fewer than five fits and only 8% having > 20 seizures. The EEG shows centrotemporal spikes on the contralateral side to the seizures. Many patients may not warrant treatment, but if it is necessary, carbamazepine or sodium valproate is effective. The seizures cease and the EEG normalizes after puberty with no enhanced risk of epilepsy in later life.

■ Juvenile myoclonic epilepsy (JME)

This is an important condition which often goes unrecognized for many years[14] as patients do not report their symptomatology on awakening; this is the hallmark of the condition. This hallmark is the presence of myoclonic jerks, usually on waking, typically involving the limbs – abduction/flexion of the shoulders and flexion of the elbows together with flexion of the hips and knees. In contrast to all other generalized seizures, consciousness is usually retained, at least during the episodes of myoclonic jerking. The jerks may occur singly, in short bursts or repeatedly with a crescendo culminating in a tonic–clonic seizure. Some 80–90% of people with JME have tonic–clonic seizures and absences occur in 30–50% of patients.

There is a strong genetic predisposition in JME, with

epilepsy occurring in near relatives in 25–50% of cases. Current thinking is that JME is an autosomal recessive condition with the gene for this condition believed to be on chromosome 6. It usually commences first in adolescence, but may occur earlier in childhood and also well into adult life.[15] Most patients have seizures shortly after waking, either in the morning or after a nap during the day. In some cases, physiological awakening during the night can provoke seizures. Thus nocturnal seizures do not exclude the diagnosis of JME. In 80–90% of cases, seizures are provoked by lack of sleep and/or alcohol ingestion the evening before. Some patients may exhibit premenstrual exacerbations, but clinical photosensitivity is uncommon. The EEG most often shows generalized irregular paroxysms with spikes and polyspikes followed by slow waves in the frequency range of 3–6 Hz. These features are seen in about 95% of untreated patients and 30% of sodium valproate-treated patients.

Management of JME consists of the use of sodium valproate, which is largely specific for this condition. Complete control can be expected in over 90% of cases. Relapses are usually related to drug non-compliance, stress, sleep deprivation and alcohol consumption.[16] In view of the likelihood of relapse on withdrawal of medication, therapy is lifelong. Patients who do not respond to valproate or develop unacceptable side effects seem to do well on lamotrigine.[17,18]

Epilepsy with GTCS on awakening

This condition is quite common with onset in adolescence (peak 14–16 years). In 30% of girls who develop it, it commences in association with their first menses. Seizures are tonic–clonic in nature and occur within an hour of waking but without the myoclonus of JME. Sleep deprivation and alcohol are strong seizure-provoking factors, with photosensitivity and a family history of epilepsy being quite common. Sodium valproate is the drug of choice with carbamazepine second choice. Most patients should be fully controlled and require treatment for 10–15 years to minimize the risk of relapse.[19]

There are naturally many more types of epilepsy that exist, but they are rare and do not warrant discussion in this particular text.

2 The aetiology, epidemiology and prognosis of epilepsy

With improved investigational techniques, a cause for epilepsy is being found in more patients than has previously been the case. Despite this, no specific cause may be found in some 60% of patients. The clinical history remains important, with particular attention being paid to the perinatal history and subsequent development, prolonged febrile convulsions, head injuries, a family history of epilepsy, previous meningitis/encephalitis or the onset of neurological symptoms. Epilepsy (recurrent seizures) is a symptom (sign) of an underlying problem and can be associated with any form of cerebral pathology which is in part age related (**Figure 1**).

In epilepsy, cortical neurones show abnormalities of membrane potential and firing patterns. The paroxysmal depolarization shift (PDS) is an abnormally large, prolonged depolarizing post-synaptic potential, which may cause the burst firing of neurones and may subsequently excite other neurones to behave similarly. The PDS can result from an imbalance between excitatory neurotransmitters (aspartate and glutamate) and/ or inhibitory neurotransmitters (GABA related) or

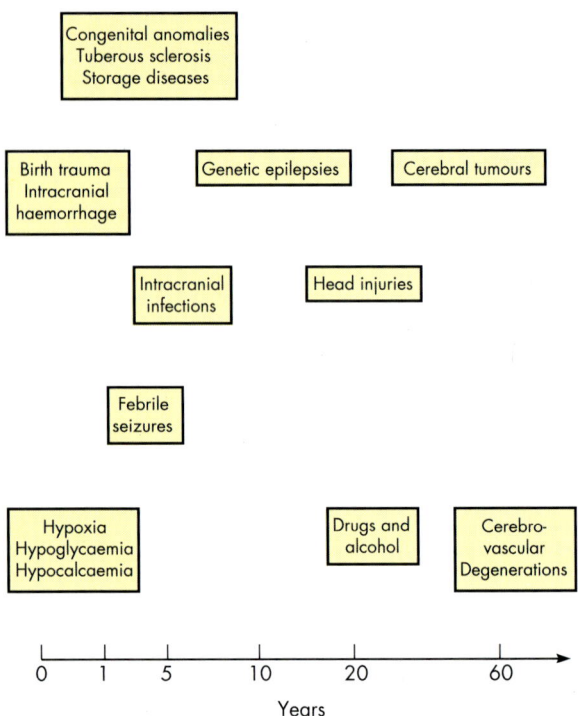

Figure 1 Causes of seizures and epilepsy by age (Reproduced, with permission, from *Medical Neurology*, Eds: Chadwick D, Cartlidge N & Bates D. Churchill Livingstone, Edinburgh, 1989)

abnormalities of voltage-controlled membrane ion channels. In primary generalized seizures, spike–wave activity is generated in cortical structures with rapid spread of recurrent excitation (spikes) and inhibition (slow waves) to the whole of both hemispheres via a corticoreticular cortical loop. In focal epileptogenesis

The aetiology and epidemiology of epilepsy

(partial seizures) there is an epileptic focus containing a group of neurones which exhibit abnormal burst firing. The extent of neuronal involvement determines the extent of the seizure.

Seizures, rather than epilepsy, may be provoked by a number of systemic problems including:

- electrolyte imbalance – hyponatraemia and hypernatraemia
- system failures – kidney, liver or respiratory
- prescribed drugs (in large doses), e.g. penicillin, theophylline, antihistamines
- drugs of addiction
- alcohol withdrawal.

These "provoked" seizures may not indicate epilepsy and rarely warrant long-term AED treatment.

As epilepsy is a condition associated with some degree of stigma and because the exact definition of epilepsy (recurrent seizures, i.e. precisely how many?) varies from study to study, accurate epidemiological data are difficult to obtain. Overall, about 1 in 20 of the population will have a seizure at some time in their lives and conservatively 1 in 200 will have epilepsy.[20] Incidence peaks for epilepsy are in the early childhood and over the age of 65 years.

Other epidemiological data pertain to outcome and the problem of recurrence after a first seizure:

Outcome

In two longitudinal studies, 20 and 15 years after the onset of epilepsy, 42%[20] and 47%[21,22] of patients had gone into remission within a year of diagnosis. The longer the seizures remain uncontrolled, the less are the chances of subsequent remission. In the Tonbridge study,[22] it was also observed that 65% of the study population had epilepsy which continued for less than 5 years followed by remission (two years seizure free) without subsequent relapse; 13% went into remission but relapsed and 22% had epilepsy which never remitted. As suggested by Shorvon[20], this strongly suggests that there are two broad forms of epilepsy:

- one group (the majority) with a mild, short-lived condition
- the other group (about 30% of the epileptic population) have a condition which is chronic with persistent seizures.

The patients with a poorer prognosis, falling into the chronic group, include people with diffuse cerebral disorders, partial or mixed seizures, progressive neurological disorders, early-onset seizures or particular syndromes, e.g. LGS, West syndrome. Further, the more difficult seizures are to control, the worse the outlook.

This begs the question about whether early treatment affects prognosis. Sufficient to say that at the present time this question has not yet been answered. This is probably because the majority of patients have mild epilepsy which responds readily to treatment. Answering the question would require identifying the "chronic" group at the outset and then seeing if early treatment affected the outcome – a difficult study to conduct.

Recurrence after a first seizure

Traditional teaching states that a single seizure does not constitute a diagnosis of epilepsy and thus should not be treated. It is suggested that this view still pertains, but it is now apparent that recurrences are more common than was previously thought. A number of studies have shown recurrence rates of 71%[23], 67%[24] and 82%.[21,22] Whilst second seizures are common, in most individuals the total number of seizures is small and epilepsy short-lived.[22] However, it might be logical to consider early treatment in individuals in whom it is highly likely that recurrences will occur, such as people with brain damage and neurological deficits.

3 Making the diagnosis

The diagnosis of epilepsy, despite advances in investigational techniques, remains largely a clinical one. It is well established that a proportion of people presenting with a possible diagnosis of epilepsy do not have the condition.[25] If in doubt about the diagnosis, wait. It is most unusual for harm to come from waiting, much less so than from inappropriately applying the label of epilepsy with its potential social implications.

The first step is to get the best possible description of the episode(s), bearing in mind that the onlookers may have been shocked or frightened at the time and will not have observed as much as you may have hoped for. GTCS are the easiest to describe, with other seizure types being more difficult. In the latter cases, onlookers find it especially difficult to assess the individual's level of consciousness or awareness, which is important in assessing whether seizures are partial or generalized.

Based on the history, the next step is to ask, "Is it epilepsy?" There is an extensive differential diagnosis which is in part age related (**Table 4**). Again, if in doubt, wait and allow the situation to develop.

If a diagnosis of epilepsy is made it is important to ask, "What kind of epilepsy?" Some cases may be obvious on the history, e.g. BFE or JME. Others will need further investigation for specific diagnosis. This step of making a precise diagnosis is important for several reasons. Firstly, it will allow the prognosis to

Making the diagnosis

> **Psychogenic episodes**
> Pseudo-epileptic seizures
> Hyperventilation
> Panic attacks
>
> **Syncopal episodes**
> Reflex syncope – postural, micturition, cough and Valsalva
> Cardiac syncope – aortic stenosis, tetralogy of Fallot, arrhythmias
> Transient ischaemic attacks
> Migraine
> Narcolepsy
> Hypoglycaemia
> Dystonic movements (young children)
> Rage attacks
> Behaviour disturbances
> Breath-holding attacks
> Benign paroxysmal vertigo
> Rigors
> Tetany
> Night terrors

Table 4 Some of the conditions which may be mistaken as seizures

be defined; secondly, it may affect the choice of treatment; finally, the patient (or parent) will know precisely what they have and thus its implications. In the great majority of situations, it is unacceptable for patients simply to have "epilepsy" in a generic sense. They need to be aware that they have complex partial seizures, JME or whatever.

■ Neurological examination

Whilst neurological examination is frequently normal in patients with epilepsy, a full examination should be conducted. Cutaneous stigmata (e.g. tuberose sclerosis, neurofibromatosis) should be sought, as well as neurological abnormalities and especially in young children, development should be assessed.

EEG

The main investigation is electroencephalography (EEG). This may not always be truly diagnostic but:

- adds weight to the clinical diagnosis
- assists in classifying the epilepsy
- may suggest an underlying structural lesion.

As stressed by Chadwick,[26] "routine interictal EEG recording is one of the most abused investigations in clinical medicine and is unquestionably responsible for great human suffering". The main misunderstanding occurs when the EEG is used to "rule out" the diagnosis of epilepsy. Between 10 and 15% of the population have an "abnormal" EEG and may be wrongly diagnosed as having epilepsy. Further, some 35% of interictal EEGs of patients with epilepsy consistently show epileptiform discharges, 50% do only with repeated EEGs and 15% never do. A single routine EEG is likely to show an epileptiform abnormality in about 50% of patients with definite epilepsy.[27] These figures do not mean that the EEG is a "bad test", but has real limitations which need to be appreciated. The EEG report always has to be interpreted in an appropriate clinical context.

Other EEG techniques include:

1. Sleep-deprived EEG: This means ensuring the patient is tired when presenting for the EEG, so that they will sleep during the test. This enhances the chances of detecting epileptiform abnormalities.
2. Video-EEG telemetry (VEEG): This technique allows concomitant recording of the EEG with

video observation so that a seizure can be seen and recorded. This is of use in particular situations:

- confirming the episode is in fact a seizure
- possible pseudo-epileptic seizures
- defining the seizure type
- as part of pre-surgical investigation.

Neuro-imaging

In the main, neuro-imaging in epilepsy means computed tomography (CT) scanning, although magnetic resonance imaging (MRI) plays an increasingly important role for "routine" neuro-imaging, as in primary generalized epilepsy the return is very low. The greatest return is in those with partial seizures. *A good working guide is focal seizures plus focal EEG features plus focal neurological signs = a definite indication for CT or MRI scanning*. Many of the lesions detected will be atrophic, but with ageing, tumours and cerebrovascular lesions become more frequent. An algorithm for the selection of patients for CT or MRI scanning is shown in **Figures 2** and **3**. In patients where it is suspected that there may be congenital cerebral abnormalities, abnormal tissue migration or when epilepsy surgery is a possibility, MRI scanning is much more useful than CT (**Figure 4a,b,c**).

Other tests include single photon emission computed tomography (SPECT) and positron emission tomography (PET). These procedures detect changes to regional blood flow and cerebral metabolism. Focal epileptogenic lesions are hypometabolic between seizures and hypermetabolic during seizures. Both tests are particularly useful when epilepsy surgery is being considered and of course have research potential.

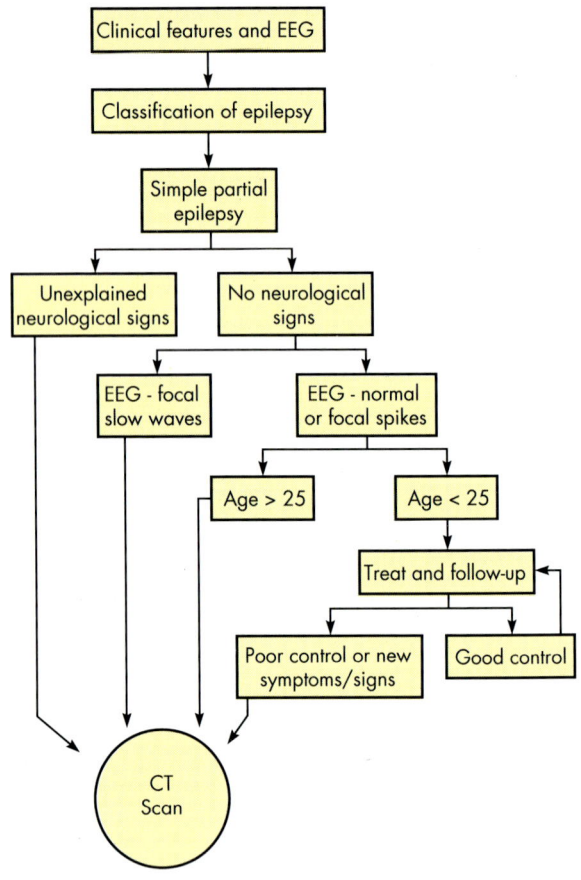

Figure 2 Guidelines for the use of CT scanning in patients with simple partial seizures
(Reproduced with permission, from *Medical Neurology*, Eds Chadwick D, Cartlidge N and Bates D. Churchill Livingstone, Edinburgh 1989)

Making the diagnosis

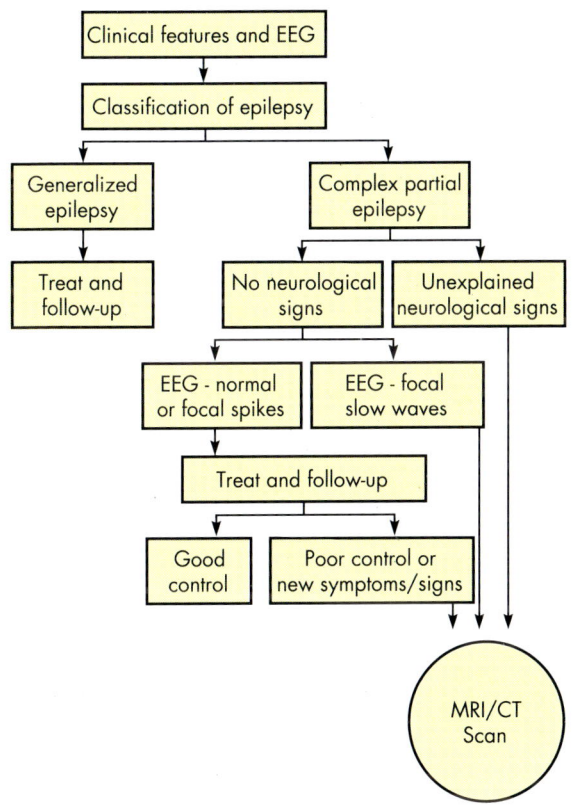

Figure 3 Guidelines for CT or MRI scanning in patients with complex partial seizures
(Reproduced, with modification and permission, from *Medical Neurology*, Eds Chadwick D, Cartlidge N and Bates D. Churchill Livingstone, Edinburgh, 1989)

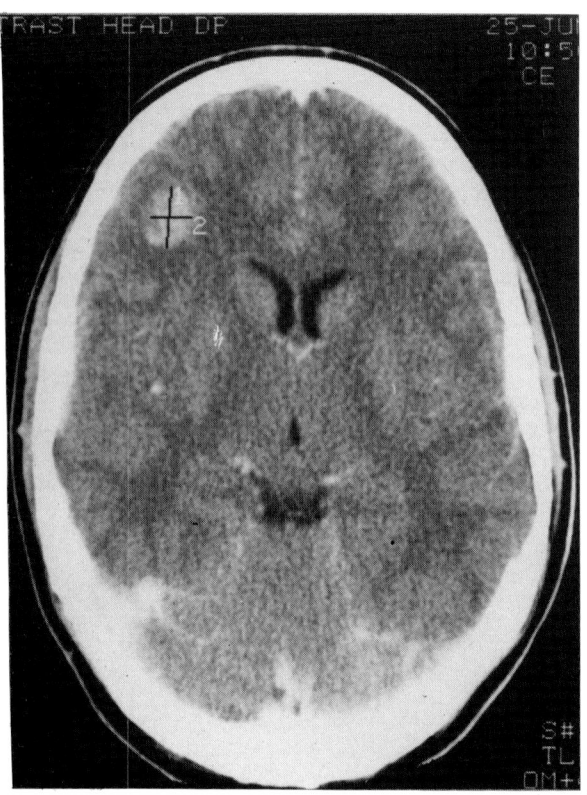

Figure 4(a) CT scan of a young man with complex partial seizures and a right frontal lobe lesion

Making the diagnosis

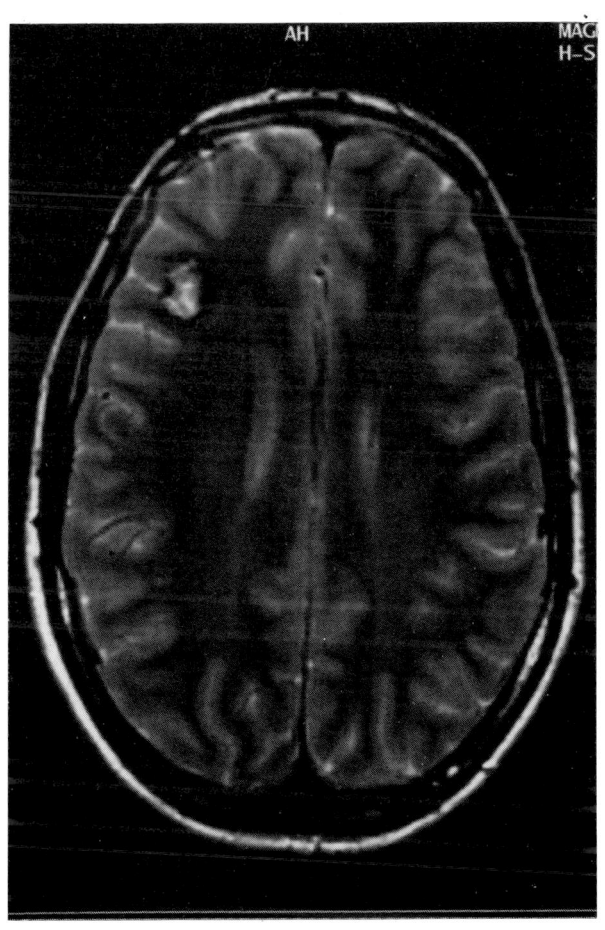

Figure 4(b) An MRI scan of the same lesion as in Figure 4(a)

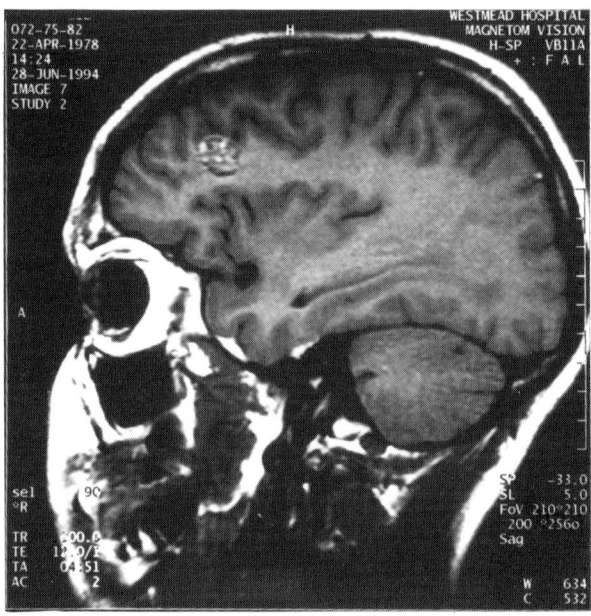

Figure 4(c) A further MRI scan of the same lesion felt as in Figure 4(a) to be a congenital venous malformation

Blood tests

There are no "routine" blood tests in the diagnosis of epilepsy. However, blood glucose and calcium should be done in young children with seizures and in certain paediatric situations much more detailed metabolic investigations may be appropriate. Investigations should be based on the clinical situation.

4 Medical management

The term "management" is again used specifically to emphasize that there is more to be considered than solely "treatment", a word usually associated with pill-taking. Nevertheless, the mainstay of management is the use of AEDs. Prior to discussing the various medications, there are several general points to be discussed.

AEDs: general points

When should AEDs treatment be commenced?

As already suggested, a single seizure would not warrant treatment but recurrent seizures would. However certain factors may suggest, on a common sense basis, a need to treat after a single seizure:

- progressive cerebral disorders
- established neurological deficits
- a clearly epileptic EEG (except in benign focal epilepsy of childhood where treatment may not be required).

In other words, situations where recurrences are highly likely.

By the same token, certain factors militate against commencing treatment:

Medical management

- seizures widely separated in time, such as annual seizures
- a previous history of non-compliance with medication
- provoked seizures – alcohol, drugs and some reflex stimuli; these are best avoided, if possible, rather than taking AEDs
- patient/parental opinions

How should AEDs treatment be commenced?

The choice of AED should be based on type of seizure or epilepsy. It has been proposed by Richens and Perucca that,[28] if there is doubt about which AED to use, sodium valproate is the most logical choice, as it has the broadest spectrum of the commonly used AEDs.

Having chosen an AED, it should firstly be used on its own (monotherapy) and the dose built up slowly over 2–4 weeks assessing efficacy by seizure control on one hand and side effects on the other. Rarely does an AED need to be introduced rapidly. Rapid introduction is often associated with side effects such as drowsiness and nausea which encourage non-compliance. Further, the rapid introduction of lamotrigine and possibly carbamazepine, may be associated with the development of a rash.

If the first AED is not successful, a second AED should be added and *the first one withdrawn* after the patient is settled on the second drug. About 30% of patients with epilepsy will need to be on more than one AED (polytherapy).

How long should treatment last and when should it stop?

This is an important issue which needs to be discussed with the patient/parents at the outset of treatment. The diagnosis of epilepsy may in itself be a shock, let alone the prospect of taking medication for an indefinite period of time. Further, all AEDs have side effects, including those of a cognitive nature, making it desirable not to treat for longer than necessary. Sadly, however, it is not possible to define the ideal length of treatment. The advice offered to patients varies widely and reflects individual clinical practice.

The first goal of treatment, of course, is to achieve seizure freedom. If this is not achieved, ceasing treatment may not be an option. As a general guide, it is suggested that:

- in primary generalized epilepsy, a one- to three-year seizure-free period is recommended
- in partial seizures, because of a higher relapse rate with medication withdrawal, a five-year seizure-free period may be desirable in adults and two to four years in children.

There is a tendency to try to withdraw AEDs earlier in children than adults because of the general concern about the effects of AEDs on the developing brain. A more conservative approach may be appropriate in adult patients because of the need to drive and to maintain employment. Social variables are important in the decision to cease treatment and patients should never be encouraged to do so against their will.

Despite the lack of precision about this decision, there are many factors which support or militate against the decision to come off treatment. These are shown in **Table 5** and are not absolute for any one individual. An abnormal EEG at the time of proposed AED withdrawal implies a greater chance of relapse, whilst a normal EEG is at best reassuring. As JME is almost always a life-long condition, drug withdrawal is almost invariably associated with relapse.

Medical management

Positive factors	Negative factors
Neurodevelopmentally normal	Neurodevelopmental deficits
Childhood epilepsy	Late-onset epilepsy
Primary generalized epilepsy	Partial seizures
Seizures which came under control rapidly	Seizures which took a long time to control
Normal EEG	Abnormal EEG
Benign epilepsy syndromes	Juvenile myoclonic epilepsy
	The need to drive
	Work-related issues

Table 5 Factors involved in the decision about withdrawing anti-epileptic medication

■ How should AEDs be withdrawn?

In a word, *slowly*. Again, there are no absolute answers to this question and practice varies widely.[29] It is suggested that for people who have been on treatment for a few years, withdrawal over three to six months should be satisfactory. Longer treatment periods (between five and ten years) might suggest slower withdrawal over six to twelve months. There is rarely any urgency about coming off medication.

■ Specific anti-epileptic drugs

Before discussing individual drugs, it should be restated that *the treatment of epilepsy is a balance between seizure control and drug side effects*. The latter, rather than the former (efficacy), allow the conventional AEDs to be divided into first- and second-line agents (**Table 6**). The role of the new AEDs is not fully defined, but they have been added with general guidelines. At present they would be used largely as add-on

Form of epilepsy	First-line AEDs	Second-line AEDs	New AEDs
Generalized epilepsy:			
Absences	VPA, ESM	CLB, CZP	LTG
JME	VPA	CZP	LTG
Awakening GTCS	VPA	CBZ, PHT	
Symptomatic generalized	VPA	CLB, CZP, CBZ, PHT	LTG, FBM*
Partial epilepsy ±	CBZ, VPA	PHT, CLB, PB	GVG, LTG, GBP, TGB
secondary generalization			
Unclassified epilepsy	VPA, CBZ		LTG

Table 6 Guidelines for the choice of anti-epileptic drugs
* Due to the problem of aplastic anaemia and hepatotoxicity, the future for felbamate is presently uncertain

therapy in resistant cases. A further factor to be taken into account when choosing an AED is cost. It is important that cost effectiveness be taken into account and this in turn requires consideration of both efficacy and side effects, although this is often difficult to achieve. In general terms, first-line drugs are likely to be more cost effective, especially in terms of quality of life, as they have fewer side effects including those of a cognitive nature. The newer AEDs are all more expensive than established AEDs and as already mentioned, their role in day-to-day practice has yet to be clarified.

AED side effects can be divided into three categories:

- dose related
- acute idiosyncrasy, e.g. rash
- chronic toxicity.

Medical management

In discussing individual drugs, side effects will be listed according to these categories. It is also worth mentioning that frequency of side effects increases with the number of AEDs being taken.[30] This is a further reason for monotherapy whenever possible.

Two other factors need to be considered when choosing an AED. The first is ease of use, e.g. twice daily dosage, or few interactions. Phenytoin has saturable metabolism which produces large serum concentration elevations (and thus potential toxicity) for small dose increases and is pharmacokinetically difficult to use. The second factor, which will be discussed later in this chapter, is whether blood-level monitoring is necessary or not. Naturally patients prefer not to have blood tests if they can be avoided.

■ Commencing AED therapy:

It is most uncommon that anti-epileptic therapy needs to be initiated rapidly other than in patients presenting with very frequent seizures or in status epilepticus.

The rapid introduction of AEDs is associated with three problems:

1. Side effects are frequent, especially of a cognitive nature, with drowsiness, lethargy and a feeling of being "drugged".
2. As a result some patients are non-compliant with their medication and seizure control is not obtained. Patients are disheartened and ask, "Will I always feel like this?"
3. Certainly with lamotrigine, when used with VPA, rapid LTG introduction may be associated with a rash. This is avoided by introducing LTG slowly. There is anecdotal evidence that the rash associated with carbamazepine may also be avoided by a slow introduction of the drug.

It is suggested that AEDs be introduced over a period of four weeks, with the exception of lamotrigine (especially when used with VPA) which might be over two to three months. A practical way of approaching this is to:

1. Decide on the intended maintenance dose, whilst accepting that this may ultimately require modification.
2. Calculate a quarter of that dose and assuming that it can be adequately taken, depending on the dose form of the preparation, commence with a one-quarter maintenance dose daily (preferably at night lest there is any drowsiness) for a week. For example, if VPA were being used aiming at a maintenance dose of 1000 mg b.d., the initial dose would be 500 mg nocte.

MEDICATION FOR	Robert Hawke			Date:	16-8-94
Medication	Dose	B/fast	Lunch	Dinner	Comments
Epilim	500 mg	–	–	1	19-8-94
↓					
Epilim	500 mg	1	–	1	26-8-94
↓					
Epilim	500 mg	1	–	2	2-9-94
↓					
Epilim	500 mg	2	–	2	9-9-94

Please contact us if you have any symptoms such as: Nausea, drowsiness, hair loss or weight gain.

Telephone Numbers: (   )

Figure 5 A patient information sheet for initiating AED therapy and providing information on common side effects

Medical management

3. This would be followed by:

   Week 2 – 500 mg b.d.
   Week 3 – 500 mg mane and 1000 mg nocte.
   Week 4 – 1000 mg b.d.

4. It is useful to provide the patient with this information in writing (**Figure 5**). Side effects should be discussed and the more frequent side effects may be added to the dosage sheet.

Whilst this approach may appear to be unduly slow, it almost totally avoids initial side effects.

Carbamazepine (CBZ)

Trade name: Tegretol.

Slow release preparation – Tegretol CR (Australia) Tegretol SR, Tegretol (Divitabs), Tegretol Retard elsewhere.

Mechanism of action: Limits repetitive firing of sodium-dependent action potentials.

Indications:
  Partial seizures – simple and complex.
  Generalized tonic–clonic seizures.

Maintenance dosage range:
  Adults: 300–1600 mg/day.
  Children: 10–40 mg/kg/day.

Dosage interval: 8–12 hourly. Slow-release, 12 hourly.

Therapeutic range: 17–42 µmol/l (4–10 mg/l). Not very useful.

Interactions: Induces the metabolism of the oral contraceptive pill, corticosteroids, haloperidol, theophylline and warfarin. CBZ metabolism is inhibited, leading to CBZ toxicity, by erythromycin, danazol, cimetidine diltiazem, isoniazid, verapamil and viloxazine.

Particular issues: Hepatic enzyme inducer. Induces its own metabolism (auto-induction), which may lead to a fall in the blood level in the first three months of treatment and may be associated with breakthrough seizures.

Side effects:
  Dose related: Double vision, dizziness, ataxia, nausea and vomiting.
  Acute idiosyncrasy: Rash, leucopenia.
  Chronic toxicity: Hyponatraemia – usually of no clinical significance, but occasionally may produce peripheral oedema and cerebral oedema (manifested by confusion and increased seizures).

Medical management

■ Clobazam (CLB)

Trade name: Frisium.
Indications: Adjunct therapy in resistant seizures.
Mechanism of action: Enhances GABA-mediated inhibition.
Maintenance dosage range:
  Adults: 10–40 mg/day.
  Children: 5–20 mg/day.
Dosage interval: Single night-time dose or 12 hourly.
Therapeutic range: Not applicable.
Interactions: None of note.
Particular issues: Tolerance occurs in about 20–40% of patients.
Side effects:
  Dose-related: Drowsiness, depression, irritability, weight gain, and in young children, drooling.

Clonazepam (CZP)

Trade name: Rivotril.
Indications: Status epilepticus, resistant absences, myoclonus and GTCS.
Mechanism of action: enhancement of GABA-mediated inhibition.
Maintenance dosage range:
  Adults: 0.5–4 mg/day.
  Children: 0.1–0.2 mg/kg/day.
Dosage interval: 8–12 hourly.
Therapeutic range: Not applicable.
Interactions: None of note.
Particular issues: Usefulness significantly limited by tolerance which is common and side effects which are frequent and affect quality of life. CZP cessation often associated with withdrawal seizures.
Side effects:
  Dose related: Sedation, functional slowing, cognitive effects and slurred speech. In children, hyperactivity, hypersalivation and bronchorrhoea.
  Acute idiosyncrasy: Rash.

Diazepam (DZP)

Trade names: Valium, Diazemuls (UK) (IV), Stesolid (UK) (rectal solution).
Indications:
  Status epilepticus (IV)
  Prophylaxis of febrile convulsions (PR, PO).
Mechanism of action: Enhancement of GABA-mediated inhibition.
Maintenance dosage range:
  Adults: 10–40 mg IV.
  Children: 0.3–0.4 mg/kg IV.
Interactions: Do not use with respiratory depressants such as phenobarbitone.
Particular issues: Not to be used IM due to poor bioavailability.
Side effects:
  Dose related: Sedation. Respiratory depression if given as a rapid IV bolus.

Ethosuximide (ESM)

Trade names: Zarontin, Emeside (UK).
Indications: Absence epilepsy.
Mechanism of action: Uncertain.
Maintenance dosage range:
  Adults: 1–2 g/day.
  Children: 20–40 mg/kg/day.
Dosage interval: 12 hourly.
Therapeutic range: 300–700 µmol/l (40–100 mg/l). Not very useful.
Interactions: None of note.
Side effects:
  Dose related: Nausea, vomiting, abdominal pain, hiccough, headache, dizziness, lethargy, ataxia and diplopia.
  Acute idiosyncrasy: Rash, aplastic anaemia.

Medical management

■ Felbamate (FBM)

Trade name: Felbatol (not licensed in UK, Australia, New Zealand, South Africa).

Indications: Resistant partial seizures, the Lennox–Gastaut syndrome and atonic seizures (drop attacks).

NB: Due to the occurrence of aplastic anaemia and hepatotoxicity associated with felbamate use, at the time of writing, the future of this AED is uncertain.

Mechanism of action: Possibly acts at the glycine site of the N-methyl-D-aspartate (NMDA) receptor.

Maintenance dosage range:
Adults: 1200–3600 mg/day.
Children: 15–45 mg/kg/day.

Dosage interval: 12 hourly.

Therapeutic range: Not of clinical value.

Interactions: FBM reduces serum CBZ concentrations, but elevates concentrations of PHT and VPA necessitating lowering the dose of these two drugs by about 25%. PHT and CBZ induce the metabolism of felbamate. Effect on the oral contraceptive uncertain at present.

Particular issues: The interactions make the drug more difficult to use than the other new AEDs.

Side effects:
Dose related: Drowsiness, headache, nausea, anorexia, weight loss and double vision.
Idiosyncratic: Aplastic anaemia and hepatotoxicity.
Chronic toxicity: Unknown.

Gabapentin (GBP)

Trade name: Neurontin.
Indications: Resistant partial seizures.
Mechanism of action: Uncertain.
Maintenance dosage range:
   Adults: 900–3000 mg/day.
   Children: Not yet defined.
Dosage interval: 12 hourly.
Therapeutic range: Not applicable.
Interactions: None of note.
Side effects:
   Dose related: Drowsiness, dizziness, double vision, ataxia and headache.
   Chronic toxicity: Not yet known.

Medical management

■ Lamotrigine (LTG)

Trade name: Lamictal.

Indications: Refractory partial or primary generalized seizures, JME and LGS.

Mechanism of action: possibly acts at voltage-dependent sodium channels, leading to a decrease in the pre-synaptic release of glutamate.

Maintenance dosage range:
  Adults: 100–800 mg/day.
  Children: Up to 5 mg/kg/day with VPA, 10 mg/kg/day with VPA and enzyme inducers and 15 mg/kg/day with enzyme inducers alone.

Dosage interval: 12 hourly.

Therapeutic range: Not applicable.

Interactions: VPA increases LTG blood levels and may cause toxicity, including rash. LTG has a pharmacodynamic interaction with CBZ producing signs of CBZ intoxication (diplopia, ataxia and dizziness).

Particular issues: Lamotrigine needs to be introduced slowly, especially in the presence of VPA. The author's personal practice, which is very conservative, is to commence with a dose of 12.5 mg LTG every 2nd or 3rd day, increasing fortnightly to 12.5 mg daily, 12.5 mg b.d., 12.5 mg mane and 25 mg nocte, 25 mg b.d., and so on. This introduction schedule is not specifically recommended, but since using it, no rashes have occurred.

The CBZ–LTG interaction can be minimized by mentioning the possibility to parents and when it occurs, ceasing CBZ for 24 hours and recommencing at a CBZ dose 25% lower than previously.

Side effects:
  Dose related: Double vision, dizziness, ataxia, nausea and headache.
  Acute idiosyncrasy: Rash (especially when used with VPA).
  Chronic toxicity: Not yet known.

Oxcarbazepine (OCBZ)

Trade name: Trileptal.
Indications: As for carbamazepine.
Maintenance dosage:
  Adults: 600–1200 mg/day.
  Children: Not yet defined.
Dosage interval: 12 hourly.
Therapeutic range: Not clearly defined.
Interactions: The interactions described for CBZ are considerably less with OCBZ.
Particular issues: Less enzyme induction.
Side effects:
  Dose related: Similar to, but less so than, with CBZ.
  Acute idiosyncrasy: Rash less frequent than with CBZ.
  Chronic toxicity: Hyponatraemia probably more common than CBZ biochemically, but probably not of greater clinical significance.

Medical management

Phenobarbitone (PB)

Trade names: Gardenol (UK), Luminal (UK), Prominal (UK, Aus).

Indications: Partial, generalized and tonic seizures, status epilepticus and the prophylaxis of febrile convulsions.

Mechanism of action: enhances GABA-mediated inhibition.

Maintenance dosage range:
  Adults: 60–240 mg/day.
  Children: 4–5 mg/kg/day.

Dosage interval: 12 hourly.

Therapeutic range: 40–172 µmol/l (10–40 mg/l). Not very useful.

Interactions: Complex interactions with other AEDs due to enzyme induction.

Particular issues: A second-line drug, because of its side effects. A potent enzyme inducer. However, it is inexpensive and thus remains an important drug in developing countries.

Side effects:
  Dose related: Drowsiness, ataxia. In children, aggression, hyperactivity and insomnia.
  Acute idiosyncrasy: Rash, hepatotoxicity, Stevens–Johnson syndrome.
  Chronic toxicity: Folate deficiency, impotence, tolerance, habituation, osteomalacia, cognitive problems and poor memory.

Phenytoin (PHT)

Trade names: Dilantin (Aus), Epanutin (UK).

Indications: Partial and generalized seizures and status epilepticus.

Mechanism of action: Inhibits sustained repetitive firing effects on sodium-dependent voltage channels.

Maintenance dosage range:
  Adults: 200–600 mg/day.
  Children: 5–8 mg/kg/day.

Dosage interval: 24 or 12 hourly.

Therapeutic range: 40–80 µmol/l (10–40 mg/l). Very useful.

Interactions: Induces other AEDs, warfarin, oral contraceptives, corticosteroids, cyclosporin and theophylline. PHT metabolism is inhibited by allopurinol, amiodarone, chloramphenicol, cimetidine, imipramine, izoniazid, metronidazole and sulphonamides.

Particular issues: Saturable kinetics make PHT difficult to use.

  In addition, side effects are such as to make PHT a second-line drug.

Side effects:
  Dose related: Drowsiness, ataxia, double vision and slurred speech.
  Acute idiosyncrasy: Rash, lymphadenopathy and hepatitis.
  Chronic toxicity: Gum swelling, acne, hirsutism, coarsened facial features, folate deficiency, osteomalacia, cognitive impairment and depression.

Medical management

■ Primidone (PRM)

Trade name: Mysoline.
Indications: Partial and generalized seizures.
Mechanism of action: Enhances GABA-mediated inhibition.
Maintenance dosage range:
  Adults: 500–1500 mg/day.
  Children: 10–30 mg/kg/day.
Dosage interval: 8–12 hourly.
Therapeutic range: 20–55 µmol/l (5–12 mg/l). Not very useful.
Interactions: As PRM is metabolized to phenobarbitone, the interactions are similar.
Particular issues: As for PB.
Side effects: As for PB.

■ Sodium valproate (VPA)

Trade name: Epilim.
Indications: Primary generalized epilepsy, partial seizures and JME. A broad-spectrum AED.
Mechanism of action: Uncertain.
Maintenance dosage range:
  Adults: 500–3000 mg/day.
  Children: 20–50 mg/kg/day.
Dosage interval: 12 hourly.
Therapeutic range: 300–700 µmol/l (50–60 mg/l). Of almost no clinical value.
Interactions: Refer to lamotrigine profile.
Particular issues: The main concerns are about hepatotoxicity which occurs largely in children less than 3 years of age with difficult epilepsy on polytherapy and the risk of spina bifida in the foetus.
Side effects:
  Dose related: Tremor, irritability, nausea and vomiting.
  Acute idiosyncrasy: Pancreatitis, hyperammonaemia and encephalopathy and hepatotoxicity (mainly young children).
  Chronic toxicity: Weight gain, hair loss, oedema.

Medical management

■ Vigabatrin (VGB)

Trade name: Sabril.

Indications: Refractory partial seizures and West syndrome (especially associated with tuberous sclerosis).

Mechanism of action: Enzyme-activated irreversible inhibitor of GABA aminotransferase.

Maintenance dosage range:
　Adults: 2000–4000 mg/day.
　Children: 50–150 mg/kg/day.

Dosage interval: 12 hourly.

Therapeutic range: Not applicable.

Interactions: None of note.

Particular issues: Use with care in individuals with a previous history of psychiatric disturbance as psychosis has been reported in this clinical setting.

Side effects:
　Dose related: Headache, weight gain, occasional drowsiness and depression.
　Chronic toxicity: Not yet known.

Therapeutic drug monitoring (TDM)

Blood-level monitoring of AEDs was very popular in the 1980s, but it has become apparent that this has been overdone. There may be few advantages in having epilepsy, but one is that most epileptics can reasonably reliably report their seizure frequency, which when looked at as seizure control, is the end point of AED therapy. TDM, because it is easily available, has become abused. Indeed blood level results have become routine, irrespective of seizure control and have become the focal point of some consultations.

The therapeutic range is essentially a statistical concept which states that most patients taking a particular AED are reasonably well controlled with few side effects if they are within the therapeutic range. However, some patients may be well controlled or may have side effects below the therapeutic range, whilst others may need to be above the therapeutic range to obtain seizure control and may be free of side effects.

As will have become apparent in the individual drug profiles, there is little role for TDM and there is no clinical benefit in measuring blood levels for the new AEDs. Useful indications for TDM include[28]:

- when using phenytoin because of its saturable metabolism; this is especially important when establishing dosage, rather than when the patient is stabilized on the drug
- when there are signs of toxicity in patients on polytherapy and it cannot be decided clinically which is the offending agent
- during pregnancy or in the presence of renal or hepatic disease
- concerns about compliance.

Using these guidelines, TDM will be kept to a minimum for which patients will be appreciative. *There is no role for "routine" TDM.*

Medical management

■ Drug compliance

Many patients with a chronic disorder, such as epilepsy, will be non-compliant from time to time. Taking medication twice or thrice daily for years on end is boring and we are all forgetful. With epilepsy, the price for significant non-compliance is a seizure or several seizures. This is usually unpleasant and few people enjoy having seizures. Thus, in the main, most epileptics are compliant most of the time. Common reasons for non-compliance in an epilepsy clinic setting are shown in **Table 7**.

Naturally, compliance must be encouraged, but by

Forgetfulness	13
Refusal to take medication/anti-medication attitude	9
Not having sufficient seizures, or the timing of the seizures (e.g. sleep associated), which in the patient's view did not warrant taking medication	8
Poor understanding of epilepsy	7
Personality disorder in patient/parent	4
Family discord	4
Risk taking:	
Stopped medication to see what would happen	4
Stopped medication to frighten or threaten others	3
Alcohol abuse	3
Doctor–patient communication problem	2
Specifically forget/avoid midday dose	2
Medication side effects	1
Muddled doses up on one occasion	1
Told by God to cease medication	1

Table 7 The reasons for non-compliance in 42 patients from an epilepsy clinic setting.[31] In some individuals there was more than one reason for being non-compliant

the same token occasional lapses are understandable and may be regarded as normal behaviour. If you doubt this, ask yourself if you have ever finished a five- or seven-day course of antibiotics? If not, why not?

Status epilepticus

Status epilepticus can be divided into:

- convulsive status
- non-convulsive status.

Status epilepticus confined to the neonatal period
Neonatal status
Status in neonatal epilepsy syndromes

Status epilepticus confined to infancy and childhood
Infantile spasms
Febrile status epilepticus
Status in childhood myoclonic syndromes
Status in benign childhood epilepsy syndromes
Electrographic status during slow-wave sleep
Syndrome of acquired epileptic aphasia

Status epilepticus occurring in childhood and adult life
Tonic–clonic status
Absence status
Epilepsia partialis continua
Myoclonic status in coma
Specific forms of status in mental retardation
Non-convulsive simple partial status
Complex partial status

Status epilepticus confined to adult life
De novo absence status of late onset

Table 8 Classification of status epilepticus[32]

Interested readers are referred to the excellent review by Shorvon[32] whose classification is shown in **Table 8**.

■ Non-convulsive status

This represents complex partial or absence status and is relatively uncommon. As a result it will not be discussed in detail. However, the condition is important as for the affected individual it is not benign. Indeed, there is good evidence that non-convulsive status can be quite intellectually and cognitively damaging. The clinical features are often subtle with the patient simply being "less with it" than usual or frankly confused. The diagnosis is made with EEG assistance. Benzodiazepines (diazepam or clonazepam) are the most useful therapy.

■ Convulsive status epilepticus

Seizures lasting more than 30 minutes become a medical emergency and represent status epilepticus which is associated with a significant morbidity and mortality. Damage is due to cerebral ischaemia and hypoxia. Initial drugs of choice are IV diazepam, midazolam (IV/IM) or lorazepam (IV). The first two agents can be used rectally in children if IV access is difficult. A slow phenytoin infusion should also be commenced to provide longer-term AED cover. If these measures fail, pseudo-epileptic seizures should be considered and EEG studies performed. Once the diagnosis is established, barbiturate anaesthesia should be instituted.

■ Non-pharmacological matters

As already mentioned, there is more to the management of epilepsy than solely the taking of pills. These issues will be discussed in more detail in Chapters 8 and 9, but warrant brief mention here.

Sleep deprivation

Sleep deprivation is a strong seizure-provoking factor for epilepsy in all age groups. It is important for people with epilepsy to get reasonable amounts of sleep and for example, if they are anticipating a late night, to have a nap during the day. This is particularly so for those with JME, mothers with infants who wake in the night and during adolescence.

Alcohol

People with epilepsy should drink alcohol very modestly, as it will increase drowsiness and may provoke seizures. Binge drinking is especially dangerous. Alcohol and sleep deprivation is a particularly bad combination.

Photosensitivity

As already discussed, not all people with photosensitive epilepsy require AED therapy. Avoidance of photic stimuli is most important, such as sitting more than 3 metres from the television, wearing sun-glasses, avoiding some computer games, etc. Many patients who do not have true photosensitivity are aware of the condition and report rather vague light-associated problems. This misunderstanding needs to be put to rest as soon as possible.

Stress

There is little evidence that epilepsy commences as a result of stress, but there is ample evidence that stress exacerbates seizures.[33] Many patients of all age groups recognize this association. *As a general rule, stress-associated seizures do not respond to an increasing AED load.* Indeed, increasing the dose may enhance drowsiness and decrease functioning which in turn increases the stress and fuels the seizures. Stress, whatever that means to the individual in question, needs to be explored in its own right. Behavioural management techniques may be very helpful.[34]

Finally, patients may ask about "alternative" therapies either because they are anxious about the use of drugs (chemicals) or because they feel desperate with intractable seizures. There is no good evidence that homeopathy, naturopathy or osteopathy are of value in epilepsy. However there are frequent anecdotal reports of cures. It is up to each practitioner to decide how they wish to tackle these issues. The author's practice is to say that it is unproven therapy, but likely to be harmless. If the patient wishes to explore a natural therapy that is fine, but, if taking AEDs, should continue them. This approach has been developed after having said "No" to several patients, who went ahead anyway, but stopped their AEDs with unfortunate results.

5 Surgical management

There are a number of surgical procedures which are specifically applicable to epilepsy, although the number of patients suitable for surgery is limited. Patients with cerebral tumours which are associated with seizures may require surgery for the primary lesion; this is not regarded as epilepsy surgery *per se*.

■ Temporal lobe surgery

This is the most commonly performed operation in the management of epilepsy, although the number of patients who are suitable for surgery is limited. Its purpose is to remove the area of epileptogenic tissue and is applicable to individuals with partial seizures arising from the temporal lobe and to a much lesser extent, the frontal lobe.

There are a number of criteria which need to be met for temporal lobe surgery to be considered, let alone successful:

1. The site of seizure onset needs to be strictly defined by EEG techniques, MRI, SPECT and PET (if available). In general terms, it needs to be demonstrated that the seizures are arising consistently from one temporal lobe, preferably anteriorly.
2. Neuropsychological assessment is essential to

assess the functional importance of the site of seizure onset. Verbal IQ and memory are left-sided functions with performance IQ and visual memory being right sided. There may, on occasion, be some memory loss with temporal lobectomy, thus those with existing memory problems need to be carefully assessed, lest their memory be further worsened by surgery.
3. In general terms, patients over 50 years of age or with an IQ less than 70 do less well.

Patients with partial seizures which have not responded to a number of AEDs should be considered for surgery. Pre-surgical investigations will identify some patients with pseudo-epileptic seizures and also will demonstrate that in others, the seizures arise from more than one site or their origin cannot be defined. These patients would not be helped by surgery.

The procedures include anterior temporal lobectomy or selective amygdalo-hippocampectomy, if the seizure onset is in the mesial temporal structures or when contralateral memory function is borderline. Overall, the results of temporal lobe surgery are good, with 50–70% of patients becoming seizure free (perhaps with occasional auras). Naturally this will be of considerable benefit to the patient, although it is important to bear in mind that the psychological problems associated with chronic epilepsy (Chapter 8) persist. Thus social isolation and employment status for example, may change little.

■ Corpus callosotomy

This is usually a two-stage (anterior and posterior) procedure which is designed to separate the two hemispheres of the brain and limit seizure spread. The procedure is usually employed in persons with intractable tonic or atonic seizures (drop attacks). It may also be used in people with unilateral cerebral pathology with focal seizures which secondarily generalize. Overall, few patients become seizure free although about 50–60% of patients show an improvement in seizure control. This, however, is not always long lasting.

Hemispherectomy

This extensive procedure removes structurally abnormal tissue and is employed in hemimegalencephaly or congenital hemiplegia and hemianopia and the Sturge–Weber syndrome. It may be outstandingly successful in carefully selected cases.

The most common of these procedures is temporal lobectomy which has been on the increase over the past decade. This trend may slow down in the 1990s with the advent of new AEDs to which a proportion of patients with currently intractable partial seizures will respond.

Finally, and not directly related to epilepsy surgery, is the question as to the value of prophylactic AED use after supratentorial neurosurgery for non-traumatic conditions. This has become quite common practice, usually with phenytoin. However, two recent studies have shown this practice does not reduce seizures either post-operatively[35] or post-trauma.[36]

6 Epilepsy in particular situations: the neonatal period, childhood, the elderly, pregnancy, the disabled and photosensitivity

The various settings discussed in this chapter are included because they warrant, albeit relatively brief, comment on specific problems.

■ Neonatal seizures[3/]

This is rather a specialist area and is quite complex. Neonatal seizures may be difficult to diagnose and

> **Day 1**
> Hypoxia
> Hypoglycaemia
> Hyperglycaemia
> Direct drug effects
> Pyridoxine dependency
> Infections
> Severe trauma
> Intracranial haemorrhage
>
> **Days 2–3**
> Infections
> Drug withdrawal
> Developmental malformations
> Intracranial haemorrhage
> Metabolic disorders (Table 10)
> Hyperglycaemia
> Hypocalcaemia
> Sodium imbalance
>
> **> Day 4**
> Developmental malformations
> Hypocalcaemia/hyperphosphataemia (dietary)
> Hyponatraemia
> Metabolic disorders
> Infection
> Drug withdrawal

Table 9 Some of the causes of neonatal seizures

need to be differentiated from jitteriness, which is stimulus sensitive. Neonatal seizures can be classified as subtle, tonic, clonic and myoclonic. Aetiological factors are shown in **Table 9** and the metabolic causes in **Table 10**. Perusal of these tables will also suggest the sorts of investigations that would be appropriate after a full clinical assessment.

Management consists of identifying and treating conditions such as electrolyte imbalance, drug withdrawal, metabolic disorders and CNS infections. If a

Epilepsy in particular situations

> Hypocalcaemia
> Hypoglycaemia
> Hypomagnesaemia
> Hyponatraemia
> Hypernatraemia
> Hyperglycaemia
> Low pyridoxine
> Amino acid disorders
> Urea cycle disorders
> Lipid storage disorders

Table 10 Some of the metabolic causes of neonatal seizures

correctable cause is not found, pyridoxine should be given and if ineffective, AED therapy should be commenced. Drugs often need to be given parenterally so phenobarbitone or phenytoin are frequently used.

■ Childhood

Most epilepsy commences in childhood so there are a number of particular issues that pertain to children with epilepsy:

1. AED doses. Children metabolize AEDs more rapidly than do adults and thus may require relatively higher doses on a mg/kg/day basis than adults.
2. Not surprisingly, children do not enjoy venipunctures for blood-level monitoring. This should be taken into account when selecting an AED.
3. Young children may not be able to describe AED side effects (dizziness, double vision, etc.) so suggestive symptoms/signs need to be sought. Cognitive side effects are also more difficult to ascertain and remain a concern with long-term AED therapy.
4. Because of these concerns, it is usual to try to

withdraw AEDs in children as soon as possible; usually after having been seizure free for about two years.
5. Parental information and education is essential (Chapter 10).
6. It is important for children with epilepsy to lead as normal lives as possible. Clearly this will depend on seizure frequency, the nature of the seizures, parental reactions and so on. This will be further discussed in Chapter 9.
7. About 15% of girls and 50% of boys with epilepsy have some form of learning difficulty, most often manifested as problems with reading, writing and arithmetic. This may relate in part to the seizures and the AEDs, but importantly may relate to the type of epilepsy (especially temporal lobe) or may be innate in the child.[38]

■ The elderly

Epilepsy in elderly persons is under-recognized, both diagnostically and in terms of its impact on social functioning. Some issues of importance include:

1. Frequency. This is uncertain due to diagnostic difficulties, but it is estimated that there are about 16 new cases per 100,000 of the population per annum in adult life, increasing to 50 per 100,000 over the age of 60 and to 75 per 100,000 over 70 years of age. The commonest times for seizures to occur are in the first year of life and old age.
2. Aetiology. Not surprisingly, the commonest cause is cerebrovascular disease followed by tumours (primary or secondary). About 25% of cases remain unexplained.[39]
3. Problems with diagnosis. Clinically, this is not always easy with the wide differential diagnosis of

Epilepsy in particular situations

"funny turns". The EEG is more difficult to interpret in the elderly and CT scans may often show abnormalities which do not relate to the epilepsy or alter management.

4. Drug therapy. The principles are the same as in other age groups, although because of the underlying aetiology in the elderly, recurrences seem likely, almost suggesting treatment after a single seizure. However, because the diagnosis is not always absolutely certain, and the elderly suffer more drug side effects (especially cognitively) and are more likely to be non-compliant with medication, a wait and see policy is often adopted.[40]

5. Social impact.[41] Epilepsy in old age is associated with physical injury (e.g. fractured hips), loss of self-confidence, fear, loss of independence and social isolation. These problems should not be under-estimated and are best assessed by home visits and family interviews.

■ Pregnancy

This important topic will be discussed briefly; interested readers are referred to Crawford[42] and Delgado-Escueta et al.[43]. The factors to be considered are shown in **Table 11(A)**.

■ Inheritance

There is a risk, at least five times greater than in the general population, that epilepsy will occur in the children born of parents, where one or both, have epilepsy. This does not apply to those with post-traumatic epilepsy.

A. The inheritance of epilepsy
   The effect of pregnancy on seizure control
   The effect of epilepsy on the pregnancy
   The teratogenicity of AEDs
   Breast feeding

B. An increased volume of distribution due to placental, uterine and foetal growth
   A decrease in plasma protein drug binding
   An increase in renal AED clearance
   An increase in hepatic AED metabolism
   Placental AED metabolism

Table 11 The major issues to be considered in pregnant epileptic women (A) and the reasons why AED blood levels may fall (B)

Effect of pregnancy on seizure control

About 50% of women will show no change in seizure frequency, 35% a deterioration and 15% an improvement. The deterioration in seizure control is probably due to AED pharmacokinetic changes and non-compliance. It is difficult to predict which patients will deteriorate, although those with difficult seizure control prior to pregnancy are more likely to be affected.

It has long been known that blood AED concentrations may fall during pregnancy for a number of reasons (**Table 11(B)**). Blood-level monitoring is thus of value, although whether this should be done routinely is unclear. Most patients will show a decrease in blood levels, but only about one-third have a deterioration in seizure control.

Effects of epilepsy on the pregnancy

There is no clear association between obstetric complications and seizure frequency. An increased bleeding

Epilepsy in particular situations

tendency in the neonate has been reported, especially with exposure to phenytoin and phenobarbitone. Vitamin K should be given to the mother prior to delivery and to the newborn infant.

Teratogenicity

This is the matter of great concern to parents and should be discussed prior to pregnancy whenever possible, especially as about 50% of epileptic mothers first present at 6–12 weeks of gestation.

Neonatal malformations occur two to three times more often in the offspring of epileptic mothers taking AEDs than in the general population. This is especially the case where there is poor seizure control and polytherapy. Abnormalities consist of minor and major congenital abnormalities, some degree of growth retardation and developmental delay. Abnormalities have been reported with all the AEDs and spina bifida occurs in 1–2% of pregnancies where sodium valproate is used. Spina bifida has also been reported with exposure to carbamazepine. Folic acid 0.5–5 mg/day should ideally be given for a month before and throughout the pregnancy to minimize this risk. Little is known at present as to the teratogenic potential of the new AEDs.

Breast feeding

All the AEDs get into breast milk to some degree, but rarely cause any clinical problems. It is fine to breast feed.

Persons with disabilities

Persons with brain damage (e.g. cerebral palsy, post-meningitis and those with intellectual handicap) have a high incidence of epilepsy. Quite commonly they have a variety of seizure types and seizures may be difficult to control. There are a number of problems in this group of patients:

1. Seizure control is often difficult leading to polytherapy and potential side effects.
2. Side effects are more difficult to assess because the patients may not be able to describe them. Parents and carers should report drowsiness, hypersalivation or drooling, ataxia or aggressive behaviour.
3. Because of the difficulty in assessing side effects, blood-level monitoring for appropriate drugs may be of greater value than in non-handicapped persons.
4. Pseudo-epileptic seizures are not uncommon and should be thought of when seizure control is difficult.
5. Because of the underlying problem of a "permanent seizure focus", AED therapy is likely to be long term and because the relapse rate on ceasing therapy is high, perhaps life-long.

With the progressive de-institutionalization of these individuals, care is more and more provided in the community, and it is important to be aware of these problems. Sedative drug therapy (e.g. benzodiazepines and barbiturates) should be avoided. Sodium valproate and lamotrigine,[7] broad-spectrum AEDs, seem to be the drugs of choice.

■ Photosensitivity

This topic has been included as a brief section in its own right, for as already mentioned, many patients

Epilepsy in particular situations

without true photosensitivity perceive light stimuli to be a factor in provoking their seizures.

About 3% of patients with epilepsy have visually induced seizures. This is most commonly seen in childhood and juvenile absence epilepsy and juvenile myoclonic epilepsy. It is much less common in symptomatic generalized epilepsies and is rare in partial seizures. The stimuli include flickering or flashing lights and pattern sensitivity (television). Photosensitivity responds well to sodium valproate and may disappear spontaneously at about 24 years of age, or earlier if controlled by VPA at an early age.

The potential of computer games to cause seizures is a topical issue and a common parental question. There is a risk, albeit small, which can be minimized by:

- not sitting too close to the screen
- not having a very bright display
- avoiding continuous exposure to the same pattern
- not playing when tired.

7 Pseudo-epileptic seizures

Pseudo-epileptic seizures (PES) occur in people with, and without, epilepsy. The frequency of PES is unclear and will vary from centre to centre depending upon the pattern of their referrals. The incidence of PES in the community is unknown.

PES represent non-epileptic seizures of a psychic nature which occur subconsciously. They occur at any age, including children (rare less than 8 years of age), but are most frequent in adolescence and early adult life, especially in women. Importantly, they also occur in individuals with intellectual handicap, contrary to the myth that "they are not capable of having PES".

Patients with PES exhibit a number of features which are similar to either their own epileptic seizures (if they have epilepsy) or seizures in general. They may, however, be sufficiently different to create the suspicion of PES (**Table 12**). There are no absolute clinical criteria for the diagnosis of PES, although some cases are much more obvious than others. It is common for people with PES to show an inexorable increase in seizure frequency despite a heavy AED load. Indeed, pseudo-status epilepticus occurs, with a seemingly remarkable resistance to the effects of benzodiazepines or barbiturates.[44]

Pseudo-epileptic seizures

Feature	Epileptic seizure	Pseudo-epileptic seizure
Precipitant	Usually none	Often an emotional precipitant
Circumstances:		
in sleep	Common	rare
when alone	Common	less common
Onset	Usually abrupt. May have short aura	May be gradual with increasing emotional symptoms
Cry at onset	Common	Unusual
Vocalization	During automatism	Common during seizure
Motor phenomenon	Stereotyped. Usually both tonic and clonic phase. Clonic movements slow as seizure continues.	Variable often tonic or clonic only. Clonic components vary in amplitude and frequency during the attack and are often "flapping" or "thrashing". Pelvic thrusting
Injury	Common	Rare
Incontinence	Common	Unusual
Tongue biting	Common	Rare
Consciousness	Usually totally lost in convulsive seizures	Variable, often possible to communicate during an attack

Feature	Epileptic seizure	Pseudo-epileptic seizure
Restraint	No effect	May resist, sometimes terminates an attack
Duration of convulsion	Usually short	May be prolonged
Termination of attack	Usually short. Confusion common. Drowsiness or sleep common	May be gradual, often with emotional display. Confusion unusual drowsiness or sleep unusual

Table 12 Features which may be helpful in differentiating between convulsive pseudo-epileptic seizures and convulsive epileptic seizures

Betts[44] describes several forms of PES:

- Swoons – with eyes closed, sinking to the floor and lying still with some eyelid flickering. These may represent a subconscious behaviour to avoid unpleasant situations or memories.
- Tantrums – throwing themselves to the floor, kicking, screaming, thrashing about, perhaps biting the inside of their cheek. Quite often in this group, attempts at restraint are met with increased effort. Tantrums occur in immature and/or brain damaged individuals and probably represent frustration and unspoken anger.
- Symbolic attacks – these may commence in a lying position and include breath-holding, gasping, back arching, pelvic thrusting and thrashing of the limbs. These episodes are seen predominantly,

but not exclusively, in women who have been sexually abused.

The diagnosis of PES may be made rapidly or may take years. It should never be rushed as many patients have both epilepsy and PES. The clinical history, supplemented if possible, by observing an episode, is the mainstay of diagnosis, but VEEG telemetry is often of diagnostic assistance. Contrary to popular belief, patients with PES often do very well,[45] especially if the symptoms have not been present for too long. In most patients, with a direct approach explaining the diagnosis and variable degree of support relative to the severity and chronicity of the PES, the episodes will cease. Relapses when under stress are common and the patient should be made aware that this may occur and indeed is probably a normal response for them as an individual.

The diagnosis and management of pseudo-epileptic seizures can be both intriguing and most rewarding.

8 Psychosocial issues

As has already been mentioned, there is more to the management of epilepsy than purely seizure control. Epilepsy is a unique condition because of its very nature. The unpredictability of seizures, the loss of control over one's body and environment, the embarrassment that may be associated with a seizure and the stigma associated with the condition all go towards shaping the epileptic's view of the world. In addition, it is accepted that there is an increased incidence of anxiety, psychosis, sexual dysfunction, affective disorders, behaviour problems and psychopathology in general, in people with epilepsy.[46] This is particularly the case in those with chronic epilepsy. It is often these factors, rather than the epilepsy *per se*, which dictate how the individual functions in society. The corollary is that obtaining seizure control may not always assist social functioning. People with epilepsy find this hard to comprehend.

■ Behavioural disturbances associated with seizures

Pre-ictal behaviour changes include irritability, depression, headache, a "funny feeling" and confusion. These may last for minutes to several days[47] and disappear after the seizure. During and after the seizure there may be changes in memory, thought process and affect. There may also be automatic behaviours, illusions and delusions, especially with CPS.

Further, as pointed out by Scambler,[48] such behaviour including the very nature of a GTCS, may make onlookers see the epileptic as being "out of control" and thus "unreliable". This view may contribute to stigmatization.

Emotional disorders

Mood disorders such as anxiety and depression are common in people with chronic epilepsy. Suicide is about four times greater in people with epilepsy than in the general population and even more frequent in those with temporal lobe epilepsy.

The unpredictability of seizures is a cause for gloom. This is more of a problem for some people than others. Some individuals who have quite infrequent seizures may take days or weeks to recover emotionally from the disappointment of having a seizure. For example, there may be a fear of leaving the house lest another seizure occurs in public.

Personality

There is no evidence for an "epileptic personality" as such, but as has already been pointed out, personality problems are not uncommon. An unusual (different) personality is most often seen in those with CPS.

Again, from a social point of view, it is not uncommon for people with epilepsy to say "I want to be normal like everyone else". Their perception is that with seizure control, all will be well. Regrettably this is not always the case. In addition, some of the behaviours exhibited before, during and after seizures, militate against epileptics being seen as normal.

However, some people seeking to be "normal", have an unjustified perception of their "abnormality"; this represents felt stigma.[49]

■ Sexuality

Patients with temporal lobe epilepsy have been shown to have a higher incidence of decreased sexuality (libido) than those with generalized seizures. In addition, the psychological problems already mentioned plus unemployment and poor self-confidence may also contribute. The contribution of AEDs to this problem is uncertain, but is probably small.

■ Cognitive problems

Cognitive changes are more common in people with chronic epilepsy than those with mild epilepsy. They include problems with memory, intellect, language and learning difficulties. The commonest complaint is that of a deteriorating memory. This is a complex problem with contributing factors including seizures (clinical and sub-clinical), AEDs (especially the second-line drugs) in high dosage, brain damage, and so on.

It is important for people with epilepsy to remember that most of us have lapses of memory and use memory cues such as note pads. Patients quite often do not do this, almost as a form of denial. Recently, a patient reported that she did not use a note pad because, if she was seen doing so, people would know that she had epilepsy!

■ Fear of seizures

A fear of seizures and their consequences is quite common and often unspoken. These fears include that of actually having a seizure, possible injury, brain damage, having a brain tumour, a mental illness or dying during a seizure.[50] For many people these fears are transient, but for others they may lead to anxiety or depression, a fear of being alone and a general obsession with their health. This question of fear is uncommonly discussed with patients and is mentioned here to encourage such conversation.

■ Acceptance and stigma

These are important issues and thus will be discussed in some detail. There are two forms of acceptance pertaining to epilepsy. *There is the individual person's acceptance of their epilepsy and there is society's acceptance of someone who has epilepsy.* These issues are separate but inter-dependent. The individual who has not accepted their epilepsy is likely to have more problems in, and with, the general community.

With regard to the matter of acceptance of epilepsy by the individual, parents and the family it has already been suggested that at the time of diagnosis of epilepsy (and many other conditions) a grief reaction develops; grief for a "loss of health". This takes a number of forms over time as depicted in **Figure 6**. The stages shown will be familiar to many readers, although not everybody will go through each phase, nor will this occur at the same rate for each individual or family.

Whatever the process that people go through, the ultimate objective is *acceptance*: acceptance that they, or their child, has epilepsy and that this is part of their life in the same way that they might have asthma, a heart condition or any other ailment of a long-term nature. Understandably, no one wants to have epilepsy, or indeed anything else that causes a "loss of health" and it is not surprising that it takes a while, sometimes a very long time, for acceptance to occur. In

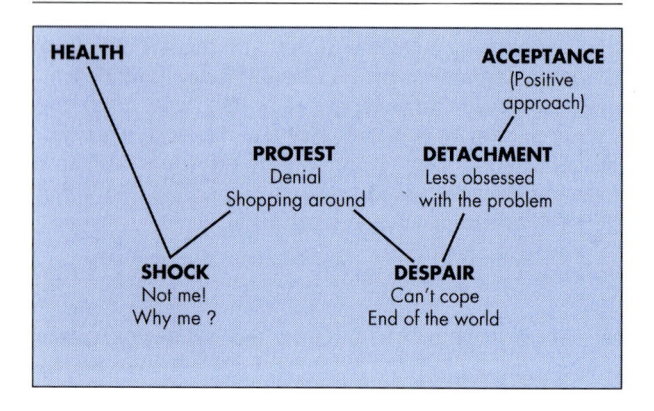

```
HEALTH                                    ACCEPTANCE
                                          (Positive
                                          approach)

              PROTEST        DETACHMENT
              Denial         Less obsessed
              Shopping around  with the problem

    SHOCK                DESPAIR
    Not me!              Can't cope
    Why me?              End of the world
```

Figure 6 A diagrammatic representation of the grief reaction which patients may undergo after the diagnosis of epilepsy

some people this never occurs, leaving them in states of anger and denial; preventing them from interacting with others and getting on with their lives. When acceptance occurs, something changes in the individual or family's life which puts their epilepsy in a different perspective. It is now only an inconvenience, or a nuisance, rather than being the central issue or the sole topic of conversation. Sometimes this is achieved, as will be discussed below, by disclosure of their epilepsy after having concealed it for years. However it occurs, it is evident to the physician and others that something has changed.

This leads to the issue of acceptance of people with epilepsy in, and by society, and the subsequent problems of discrimination and stigma. Why should society not accept people with epilepsy? According to those with the condition, there are a number of reasons:

- Public ignorance about epilepsy. Studies over the years have shown this to be less of a problem than generally perceived by people with epilepsy.

Psychosocial issues

- A view that the public is intolerant of people with epilepsy. Factually, there is little evidence to support this proposal. It may be that people are frightened by seizures, but in the main they are sympathetic. Having said this, it has to be accepted that seizures may be frightening to observe and it is difficult to convince onlookers that behaviour during a seizure is "normal". Because patients function normally between seizures, most people would never know they have epilepsy. Only when they are having a seizure ("behaving strangely") is it recognized they have epilepsy.
- A view that the public discriminates against people with epilepsy. As will be argued below, this is probably more perceived than real, but the perception continues.
- The perception that the public recognizes an epileptic "identity". Studies have certainly shown that society at large perceives people with epilepsy as "nervy", highly strung, aggressive or withdrawn. There is not, however, a general view of an epileptic "identity".

Whilst it has been shown on numerous occasions that not all people with epilepsy feel discriminated against (stigmatized), many do. The relationship between the severity of seizures and the perception of stigma has been shown to be largely dependent on other characteristics in the individual with epilepsy, such as the perception of employment discrimination, the perception of limitations imposed by the disorder and the extent of the individual's education. If stigma does exist, why should it? As proposed by Scambler,[48] it may well be that people with epilepsy threaten the social order. Why might this be?

One view is that there may be an innate prejudice against epilepsy based on a fear that the epileptic is liable to a sudden, unpredictable and sometimes dramatic loss of body control, of "going berserk". Another view is that each fit represents a loss of control which in turn implies that the individual cannot be relied upon. If they cannot be relied upon and cannot be cured, then they should be set apart (isolated). Other views include the suggestion that due to their seizures, and behaviour during them, epileptics fail to conform to cultural norms by being "imperfect". A combination of the unpredictability of epilepsy, the drama of major seizures and the fear of onlookers of having to cope with a seizure are also important factors to be considered.

Whichever of these views is held to be "correct", there is some truth (reality) in all of them. They need to be reflected upon by all of us who deal with epilepsy, but very much so by people with epilepsy who seek to understand how society sees them.

At this stage, it is useful to define the distinction drawn by Scambler between *enacted* and *felt* stigma:

- *Enacted* (real) stigma = episodes of discrimination against people with epilepsy solely on the grounds of their social and cultural unacceptability. (This excludes "legitimate" discrimination such as not being able to drive a car or fly a jumbo jet).
- *Felt* (perceived) stigma = the shame that many people with epilepsy feel and the fear of being confronted by enacted stigma. That is, the belief that people are poised, waiting to find fault and discredit the person because of their epilepsy.

The differentiation between these two forms of stigma, which could in part be called real (enacted) and perceived (felt) stigma, is extraordinarily important for people with epilepsy to appreciate. The implied difference between the terms "real" and "perceived" does not mean that "perceived" (felt) stigma is any less painful. Indeed, it will be suggested that it is

Psychosocial issues

much more frequent than "real" (enacted) stigma and equally as painful.

Bearing these distinctions in mind, it is appropriate at this point to refer to a model constructed by Scambler and Hopkins. It has been called the *hidden distress model* and has three parts:

1. When a doctor makes a diagnosis of epilepsy, the individual or the family rapidly learn to regard the status of "being epileptic" as a social liability. They adopt "a special view of the world" in which a fear of enacted stigma dominates.
2. This "special view of the world" encourages people to conceal their condition and its diagnostic label from others, in an attempt to pass as normal. That is, the fear of enacted stigma leads to a personal/family policy of "not declaring".
3. The policy of concealment[51] reduces the opportunities for enacted stigma as far as personal, family and work relationships are concerned. However, it leads to felt stigma and the ongoing (everlasting) fear of enacted stigma, disrupting people's lives more so than occasional episodes of enacted stigma.

In other words, whilst real (enacted) stigma may occur from time to time, this is likely to be quite infrequent, albeit distressing. Concealment leads to progressive perceived (felt) stigma which becomes self-perpetuating, a way of life, thereby producing ongoing pain and anguish.

In a detailed study of 24 families where a child had epilepsy, Patrick West looked at the question of concealment. Against a background of felt (perceived) stigma, he found the problem for most families was whether or not to disclose the child's epilepsy. Whilst West's studies looked solely at children and families, the principles can be applied to other age groups as well. Where seizures occur unpredictably, seemingly associated with "antisocial behaviour", concealing the condition seemed a good idea. However, concealing involves the risk of misadventure. Disclosure (declaration) means that others are at least forewarned and can avoid some of the risks associated with seizures.

Three main behaviour patterns were identified:

- *Successful concealers* – where the child's epilepsy remained unknown to almost everyone.
- *Failed concealers* – those who were, and remained, committed to concealing, despite the fact this had already failed due to involuntary disclosure or the child being seen by others during a seizure.
- *Disclosers* – those who were open about the epilepsy from the start or who failed in their attempts to conceal the problem.

Successful concealing perpetuated felt stigma as the reactions of others were never tested. If, when tested, the reactions of others were positive, rather than negative as expected, these people showed a willingness to change their views. Not testing reactions encouraged their inherent negative view. Successful concealing implies little activity outside the home and is associated with social isolation and over-protection. Failed concealers are graduates of the school of successful concealers. Put simply, their "cover has been blown". Their reaction to their "failure" was to work even harder at concealment, making it almost a way of life which caused further family problems and cemented a belief that the child was "defective" (imperfect). Only the disclosers approached normality, reinforcing the need for disclosure, if at all possible. Whilst these patterns of concealment were described in families and pertained to children, day-to-day clinical practice suggests that the same principles are applicable to all age groups.

9 Epilepsy and lifestyle

It is not helpful to provide a long list of dos and don'ts for people with epilepsy. The majority of problems can be solved with common sense, bearing in mind that most people have mild epilepsy, while others are more severely affected. There are also those people who not only have seizures but some other underlying problem which can restrict their activities. Quite obviously the person who has a seizure once a year is likely to approach life differently to someone who has a seizure once a week or several times a day. The factors that need to be taken into account are:

- the nature of the seizures
- the severity of the seizures
- when the fits occur
- the age of the patient.

When epilepsy is first diagnosed, people are often shocked and frightened. Understandably, this may lead to some degree of overprotection. However, once the seizures are controlled and an explanation and advice are provided, confidence will grow and they should be encouraged to lead as full a life as possible. There are some practical points that are worth mentioning here. These are discussed below

Specific activities

Swimming

People with epilepsy should never swim alone, and the companion should know that the person has epilepsy and what to do if a seizure should occur. *Scuba diving and springboard diving* are best avoided.

Bathing

Showering is preferable to bathing, but if the individual wishes to have a bath, they should not be left alone in the house.

Showering

The risks of showering are threefold:

- If someone has a tonic–clonic convulsion in the shower it may be difficult to get to them.
- They might push a limb through a glass panel. Showers should be fitted with the best shatter-proof glass or ideally with no glass at all, but a surrounding curtain. Wire reinforced glass is, in fact, weaker than sheet glass.
- The hot tap may be turned on fully if bumped during a seizure, resulting in burns. This may be prevented by fitting a temperature-controlled device to the water system in the shower.

Bicycle riding

The person with epilepsy who is not having frequent seizures can ride a bicycle taking the normal precautions that any other cyclist would take, including wearing a helmet.

Epilepsy and lifestyle

Horse-riding

People with epilepsy who wish to ride a horse should wear a helmet and ride with other people.

Climbing

This should probably be avoided.

Cooking

There is always concern that people with epilepsy might have a seizure whilst at the stove. For the individual with quite frequent seizures it would be wise to invest in a microwave cooker.

Sleeping

For those who have purely sleep-associated seizures, whilst the risk of suffocation during a seizure is very small, it could possibly occur. It might thus be better to have a safety pillow in the form of a firm foam pillow rather than a softer feather pillow or, in young children, perhaps no pillow at all.

Travelling

Epilepsy presents no constraint to travelling, but for individuals who have frequent seizures, it is necessary to make sensible travel arrangements. Air travel as such does not provoke seizures, but a lack of sleep on long flights and too many "free" drinks should be avoided if possible. It may be wise to provide patients with a letter about their epilepsy and their medication. Also remind them to take out travel insurance.

Driving

Driving a car has become an integral part of everyday life. Not being able to drive is at best inconvenient and may also limit job prospects. Driving regulations vary from country to country and, in Australia, from state to state. The general rules are that individuals need to be seizure free for one or two years, depending upon where they live, prior to obtaining a driving licence. In some situations where, for example, seizures occur only during sleep, the person may be allowed to drive. It is important for people with epilepsy to remember that driving a car is a responsibility and that restrictions are imposed for their own protection and for the protection of other road users. Individuals who are wishing to drive should contact their local Roads and Traffic Authority to obtain information on the current regulations for driving.

In the UK, a driving licence can be issued after the individual has been completely free of seizures (including non-convulsive seizures and auras) for one year, or free of seizures other than in sleep for three years. After ten years free from seizures and if all medication has been withdrawn, it is possible to obtain a commercial driving licence for large goods or public transport vehicles.

Employment

This may present problems for people with epilepsy. Not surprisingly, because of the nature of the condition, some occupations are simply not suitable. These would include driving a public transport vehicle, working with heavy or dangerous machinery or working at heights. Basically, two factors need to be taken into account: the possibility of sustaining an injury during a seizure and the possibility of causing harm to others.

What occupations then are not available to people with

Epilepsy and lifestyle

epilepsy? This will vary a little from country to country but, in the main, it would be unusual for an individual to obtain a post in the UK armed forces, police, fire services or in physical education teaching in schools. Other examples include occupations such an airline pilot, driving a public transport vehicle, being a crane driver and such like. It is logical, and appropriate, that people with epilepsy should not be involved in such occupations. Apart from these few exceptions, the vast majority of occupations and careers are open to people with epilepsy. Specific information is available for prospective employers and employees from the UK Employment Medical Advisory Service, and also from the Disability Employment Adviser in the local Job Centre.

10 Information for patients

As already suggested, it is important that people with epilepsy and parents know more than simply "I or my child has epilepsy". The following are suggestions as to information that patients should receive over a period of time:

- Is it epilepsy? Yes, no or unsure at present. If the last, wait for the situation to develop.
- What type of epilepsy? This needs to be defined as precisely as possible.
- What is the outlook for that type of epilepsy? For example, benign focal epilepsy of childhood will remit in adolescence, as opposed to juvenile myoclonic epilepsy which is almost always a life-long condition, albeit usually very well controlled.
- What tests are necessary? Patients need to know about each test and what it is intended to achieve.
- Is treatment needed? As already discussed, AED therapy is not always necessary.
- Which AED? The choice of a particular medication should be explained as well as common side effects.
- What medications cannot be taken with the AED? For example, erythromycin should be avoided with carbamazepine or the need for a high-dose oral contraceptive (or other form of contraception) when enzyme-inducing AEDs are being used.
- Pregnancy? All women of child-bearing age should

be provided with information on epilepsy and pregnancy.
- For how long will treatment be needed? This does not necessarily need to be absolutely precise, but people need to know if they are looking at treatment for two years, five years or for life.
- How often will blood tests be required? As already mentioned, the need for blood-level testing is relative and patients/parents should be informed of what may be required and why.
- If treatment is withdrawn after being seizure free for a time period, what will happen? This information, as discussed earlier, is not always precise, but should be openly discussed.
- What does having epilepsy imply? This needs to be talked about openly and recurrently.

These questions are based on information sought by patients and parents. There are of course many more questions which arise from time to time in particular situations. However, those mentioned above should provide sufficient information for the patient to be reasonably knowledgeable.

- What are your seizures?
- What type of epilepsy do you have?
- What tests are required?
- Is medication required?
- If so, what are the side effects?
- Can other medications be taken with the proposed anti-epileptic medications?
- Will blood tests be required?
- For how long will I need to take the medication?
- What effect will having epilepsy have on my life?

Table 13 A suggested list to give to the newly diagnosed patient to encourage them to think about their epilepsy

The author has found a summary list of these points, given to patients or parents, useful in encouraging them to think about their diagnosis and its implications **Table 13**.

References

1. Commission on Classification and Terminology of the International League Against epilepsy. Proposal for revised clinical and electro-encephalographic classification of epileptic seizures. *Epilepsia* 1981, 22, 489–501.
2. Commission on Classification and Terminology of the International League Against Epilepsy. Proposal for classification of epilepsies and epileptic syndromes. *Epilepsia* 1989, 30, 389–399.
3. Tibbles JAR. Dominant benign neonatal seizures. *Dev Med Child Neurol* 1980, 22, 664–667.
4. Bankier, A, Turner M and Hopkins IJ. Pyridoxine-dependent seizures – a wider clinical spectrum. *Arch Dis Child* 1983, 58, 415–418.
5. Chiron C, Dulac O, Beaumont D, Palacios L, Pajot N & Mumford J. Therapeutic trial and vigabatrin in refractory infantile spasms. *J Child Neurol* 1991, 6, Suppl 2, 2S52–2S59.
6. Timmings PL & Richens A. Lamotrigine as an add-on drug in the management of Lennox–Gastaut syndrome. *Eur Neurol* 1992, 32, 305–307.
7. Buchanan N. Lamotrigine – clinical experience in 93 patients with epilepsy. *Acta Neurol Scand* (in press).
8. The Felbamate Study Group in Lennox–Gastaut syndrome. Efficacy of felbamate in childhood epileptic encephalopathy (Lennox–Gastaut syndrome). *N Engl J Med* 1993, 328, 29–33.
9. Dodson WE. Felbamate in the treatment of the Lennox–Gastaut syndrome: results of a 12 month

open-label study following a randomized clinical trial. *Epilepsia* 1993, **34**, Suppl 7, S18–S24.

10. Offringa M, Derksen-Lubsen G, Bossuyt P & Lubsen J. Seizure recurrence after a first febrile convulsion: a multivariate approach. *Dev Med Child Neurol* 1992, **34**, 15–24.

11. Verity CM and Goldberg J. Risk of epilepsy after febrile convulsions: a national cohort study. *Br Med J* 1991, **303**, 1373–1376.

12. Rosman NP, Colton T, Labazzo J et al. A controlled trial of diazepam during febrile illnesses to prevent recurrence of febrile seizures. *N Engl J Med* 1993, **329**, 79–84.

13. Aicardi J. *Epilepsy in Children*. Raven Press, New York, 1986, p. 119.

14. Grunewald RA, Chroni E and Panayiotopoulos CP. Delayed diagnosis of juvenile myoclonic epilepsy. *J Neurol Neurosurg Psychiatr* 1992, **55**, 497–499.

15. Gram L, Alving J, Sagild JC, Dam M. Juvenile myoclonic epilepsy in unexpected age groups. *Epilepsy Res* 1988, **2**, 137–140.

16. Penry JK, Dean JC & Riela AR. Juvenile myoclonic epilepsy: long term response to therapy. *Epilepsia* 1989, **30**, Suppl 4, S19–S23.

17. Sharpe C & Buchanan N. Juvenile myoclonic epilepsy: Diagnosis, management and outcome. *Med J Austr* 1995, **162**, 133–134.

18. Timmings PL and Richens A. Efficacy of lamotrigine as monotherapy for juvenile myoclonic epilepsy: Pilot Study results. *Epilepsia* 1993, **34**, Suppl 2, 160.

19. Wolf P. Epilepsy with Grand Mal on awakening. In Roger J, Dravet C, Bureau M, Dreifuss FC & Wolf P (Eds). *Epileptic Syndromes in infancy, childhood and adolescence*. London, John Libbey, 1985, pp. 259–270.

20. Shorvon SD. Epidemiology, classification natural history and genetics of epilepsy. *Lancet* 1990, **336**, 93–96.
21. Annegers JF, Hauser WA & Elueback L. Remission of seizures and relapse in patients with epilepsy. *Epilepsia* 1979, **20**, 729–737.
22. Goodridge DMG & Shorvon SD. Epileptic seizures in a population of 6000. 1. Demography, diagnosis and classification. *Br Med J* 1983, **287**, 641–644.
23. Goodridge DMG & Shorvon SD. Epileptic seizures in a population of 6000. 2. Treatment and prognosis. *Br Med J* 1983, **287**, 645–647.
24. Elwes RDC, Chesterman P & Reynolds EH. Prognosis after a first untreated tonic clonic seizure. *Lancet* 1985, **2**, 752–753.
25. Buchanan N & Penna C. Non-epilepsy: a clinical perspective. *Med J Aust* 1991, **155**, 464–468.
26. Chadwick D. Diagnosis of epilepsy. *Lancet* 1990, **336**, 291–295.
27. Ajmone-Marsan C & Zivin L. Factors related to the occurrence of typical paroxysmal abnormalities in the EEG records of epileptic patients. *Epilepsia* 1970, **11**, 361–381.
28. Richens A & Perucca E. Clinical pharmacology and medical treatment. In *A Textbook of Epilepsy*, Eds Laidlaw J, Richens A & Chadwick D. Churchill Livingstone, Edinburgh, 1993, pp. 495–559.
29. Duncan JS & Shorvon SD. Rates of antiepileptic drug reduction in active epilepsy – current practice. *Epilepsy Res* 1987, **1**, 357–364.
30. Collaborative Group for Epidemiology of Epilepsy. Adverse reactions to antiepileptic drugs: a multicenter survey of clinical practice. *Epilepsia* 1986, **27**, 323–330.
31. Buchanan N. Non-compliance with medication

amongst persons attending a tertiary referral epilepsy clinic: implications, management and outcome. *Seizure* 1993, **2**, 79–82.

32. Shorvon SD. Tonic clonic status epilepticus. *J Neurol Neurosurg Psychiat* 1993, **56**, 125–134.
33. Betts T. Epilepsy and stress. *Br Med J* 1992, **305**, 378–379.
34. Fenwick P. Behavioural therapy of epilepsy. In: *Epilepsy*, Eds Pedley TA & Meldrum BS. Churchill Livingstone, Edinburgh, 1992, pp. 223–235.
35. Foy PM, Chadwick DW, Rajgopalan N, Johnson AL & Shaw MDM. Do prophylactic anticonvulsant drugs alter the pattern of seizures after craniotomy? *J Neurol Neurosurg Psychiat* 1992, **55**, 753–757.
36. Temkin NR, Dikmen SS, Wilensky AJ, Reihm J, Chobal S & Winn HR. A randomized, double blind study of phenytoin for the prevention of postraumatic seizures. *N Engl J Med* 1990, **323**, 497–502.
37. Myers GJ and Cassady G. Neonatal seizures. *Pediatr Rev* 1983, **5**, 67–72.
38. Buchanan N. Epilepsy and learning. *Aust Paediatr J* 1988, **24**, 331–333.
39. Luldorf K, Jensen LK & Plesner AM. Etiology of seizures in the elderly. *Epilepsia* 1986, **27**, 458–463.
40. Tallis R. Epilepsy in old age. *Lancet*, 1990, **336**, 295–296.
41. Ludhorf K, Jensen LK & Plesner AM. Epilepsy in the elderly: incidence, social function and disability. *Epilepsia* 1986, **27**, 135–141.
42. Crawford P. Epilepsy and pregnancy. *Seizure* 1993, **2**, 87–90.
43. Delgado-Escueta AV, Janz D & Beck-Mannagetta G. (Eds) Pregnancy and teratogenesis in epilepsy. *Neurology* 1992, **42**, Suppl 5.
44. Buchanan N & Snars J. Pseudoseizures (non

epileptic attack disorder) – clinical management and outcome in 50 patients. *Seizure* 1993, **2**, 141–146.
45. Betts T. Pseudoseizures: seizures that are not epilepsy. *Lancet*, 1990, **36**, 163–164.
46. Whitman S & Hermann BP (Eds) *Psychopathology in Epilepsy – Social Dimensions*. Oxford University Press, Oxford, 1986.
47. Hughes J, Devinsky O, Feldmann E & Bromfield E. Premonitory symptoms in epilepsy. *Seizure* 1993, **2**, 201–203.
48. Scambler G. *Epilepsy.* Routledge, London, 1989.
49. Buchanan N. *Understanding Epilepsy.* Simon & Schuster, Sydney, 1994.
50. Mittan R. Fear of seizures. In: *Psychopathology in Epilepsy – Social Dimensions*, Eds Whitman S & Hermann BP. Oxford University Press, Oxford, 1986, pp. 90–121.
51. West P. The social meaning of epilepsy: stigma as a potential explanation for psychopathology in children. In: *Psychopathology in Epilepsy, – Social Dimensions*, Eds Whitman S & Hermann BP. Oxford University Press, Oxford, 1986, pp. 245–265.

Appendix 1: Drugs in development

Piracetam. This has been used as a memory enhancer for some time, but has recently been found to have a useful antimyoclonic effect. Presently, it is in a clinical trial phase.

Tiagabine. This AED, which is available as 2, 4 and 8 mg tablets, has been shown to be effective in partial seizures.

Topiramate. This is a derivative of acetazolamide which is sometimes used in the treatment of epilepsy. Preliminary studies suggest usefulness in partial seizures.

Zonizimide. This is a drug which was shown to be useful in partial and myoclonic seizures. Development was halted as some patients developed kidney stones. The drug is presently being re-evaluated and it is likely that zonizimide will make a return to clinical trials.

Remacimide. This is showing early promise in the treatment of intractable partial seizures.

There are a number of other agents in an early stage of study.

Appendix 2: Epilepsy centres

These are units with a particular interest in epilepsy. Telephone numbers are correct at the time of going to press. However, check with your local telephone directory.

Australia

Australian Capital Territory
- Woden Valley Hospital, Woden, Canberra ACT (06 244 2222)

New South Wales
- Prince Henry Hospital, Little Bay, Sydney (02 661 0111)
- Prince of Wales Children's Hospital, Randwick, Sydney (02 399 0111)
- Royal Alexandra Hospital for Children, Camperdown, Sydney (02 519 0466)
- Royal Prince Alfred Hospital, Camperdown, Sydney (02 516 6111)
- Westmead Hospital, Westmead, Sydney (02 633 6333)

Appendix 2: Epilepsy centres

Queensland

- Royal Brisbane Hospital, Herston, Brisbane (07 253 8111)

South Australia

- Queen Elizabeth Hospital, Woodville, Adelaide (08 345 0222)

Victoria

- Austin Hospital, Heidelberg, Melbourne (03 496 5000)
- Royal Children's Hospital, Parkville, Melbourne (03 345 5522)
- Royal Melbourne Hospital, Parkville, Melbourne (03 342 7000)

Western Australia

- Royal Perth Hospital, Perth (09 224 2244)

UK

Assessment centres

- Bootham Park Hospital, Bootham, York YO3 7BY (01904 610777)
- The Centre for Epilepsy, Maudsley Hospital, Denmark Hill, London SE5 8AZ (0171 703 6333)
- Chalfont Centre for Epilepsy, Chalfont St. Peter, Bucks SL9 0RJ (01494 873991)
- David Lewis Centre, Alderley Edge, Cheshire SK9 7UD (01625 872613)
- Park Hospital for Children, Old Road, Headington, Oxford OX3 7LQ (01865 741717)

Appendix 2: Epilepsy centres

Residential centres

- Chalfont Centre for Epilepsy, Chalfont St. Peter, Bucks SL9 0RJ (01494 873991)
- David Lewis Centre, Alderley Edge, Cheshire SK9 7UD (01625 872613)
- The Maghull Homes, The Bartlett Home, Liverpool South Road, Maghull, Merseyside L31 8BR (0151 526 4133)
- Meath Home for Women and Girls with Epilepsy, Westbrook Road, Godalming, Surrey GU7 2QJ (01483 415095)
- Quarrier's Homes, Bridge of Weir, Renfrewshire PA11 3SA (01505 612224)
- St. Elizabeth's School, Much Hadham, Herts SG10 6EW (01279 843451)

Special schools for children with epilepsy

- David Lewis Centre, Alderley Edge, Cheshire SK9 7UD (01625 872613)
- St. Elizabeth's School, Much Hadham, Herts SG10 6EW (01279 843451)
- St. Piers Lingfield, St. Piers Lane, Lingfield, Surrey RH7 6PN (01342 832243)

Appendix 3: Epilepsy associations

This information is correct at the time of going to press, but may alter with time. Check your local telephone directory.

■ Australia

- Australian Capital Territory

    Epilepsy Association of the Australian Capital Territory Inc., Room 8, Fifth Floor, Royal Canberra Hospital North, Acton Peninsula, ACT 2601
    Telephone: 06 247 6267

- National Epilepsy Association of Australia

    PO Box 224, Parramatta NSW 2150
    Telephone: 02 891 6118
    Fax: 02 891 6137

- New South Wales

    Epilepsy Association of New South Wales,
    454 Pennant Hills Road,
    PO Box 343,
    Pennant Hills, NSW 2120

Appendix 3: Epilepsy associations

		Telephone: 02 980 6477
		Telephone (Community Service Centre, Parramatta): 02 891 6822
•	Queensland	Epilepsy Association of Queensland Inc., 381–385 Brunswick Street, Fortitude Valley, Qld 4006
		Telephone: 07 852 2850
•	South Australia	Epilepsy Association of South Australia Inc., 6 Woodville Road, Woodville, SA 5011
		Telephone: 08 456 131
•	Tasmania	Epilepsy Association of Tasmania Inc., 82 Hampden Road, Battery Point, Hobart, Tasmania 7004
		Telephone: 002 34 6967
		Telephone (Launceston): 003 44 0555
•	Victoria	Epilepsy Foundation of Victoria, 818–822 Burke Road, Camberwell, Vic 3124
		Telephone: 03 813 2866
•	Western Australia	West Australian Epilepsy Assoc. Inc., 14 Bagot Road, Subiaco, WA 6008
		Telephone: 09 381 1187

Appendix 3: Epilepsy associations

■ New Zealand

■ National

Epilepsy Association of New Zealand, 610 Victoria Street, Hamilton (07 834 3556)

■ Regional branches and interest groups

Auckland	14a Horoeka Avenue, Mount Eden, Auckland	09 638 7639
Central Northland	PO Box 712, Whangarei	09 438 5498
Christchurch	PO Box 2468, Christchurch	03 379 8175
Far North	PO Box 256, Kaitaia	09 408 0010 Ext 870 (hospital)
Gisborne	28 Rua Street, Gisborne	06 867 2002
Hawkes Bay	PO Box 3216, Onekawa, Napier	06 835 5537
Manawatu	Wanganui Branch, PO Box 4322, Wanganui	06 347 1081
Nelson	PO Box 2179, Stoke, Nelson	03 544 6653
Otago	PO Box 1142, Dunedin	03 477 1751
Rotorua	PO Box 1775, Rotorua	07 346 3912
Southland	PO Box 68, Invercargill	03 218 3089
Taranki	PO Box 5102, New Plymouth	06 757 8603

Appendix 3: Epilepsy associations

Taupo	Rotorua Branch, PO Box 1775, Rotorua	07 346 3912
Thames	Waikato Branch, PO Box 683, Hamilton	07 838 1433
Timaru	PO Box 3011, Timaru	03 684 7151
Tokoroa	Waikato Branch, PO Box 683, Hamilton	07 838 1433
Waikato	PO Box 683, Hamilton	07 838 1433
Wanganui	PO Box 4322, Wanganui	06 347 1081
Wellington	PO Box 44180, Lower Hutt, Wellington	04 567 5169
Whakatane	39 Brabant Street, Whakatane	07 308 4438

■ UK

- British Epilepsy Association, Anstey House, 40 Hanover Square, Leeds LS3 1BE (01345 089599)
- Epilepsy Association of Scotland, 48 Govan Road, Glasgow GS1 1JR (0141 427 4911)
- Epilepsy Association of Scotland, 13 Guthrie Street, Edinburgh EH1 1JG (0131 226 5458)
- National Society for Epilepsy, Chalfont Centre for Epilepsy, Chalfont St. Peter, Bucks SL9 0RJ (01494 873991)
- Wales Epilepsy Association, Ypant Teg, Brynteg, Dolgellau, Gwynedd LL40 1RP (01341 423339)

■ Ireland

Irish Epilepsy Association, 249 Crumlin road, Dublin 12 (3531 557500)

Appendix 4: Further reading

The following are recommended to patients with epilepsy.

Brown, R. *Young People and Epilepsy*, National Epilepsy Association of Australia, Sydney, 1993.

Chadwick, D & Usiskin, S. *Living with Epilepsy*, Methuen, Melbourne, 1987.

Epilepsy Association of Queensland. *Shadows of Discrimination: A Study of Epilepsy in Queensland*, Brisbane, 1993.

Goss, S. *Ragged Owlet*, Houghton Mifflin Australia, Melbourne, 1989.

Laidlaw, MV & Laidlaw J. *People with Epilepsy*, Churchill Livingstone, Edinburgh, 1984.

Sanders L & Thompson P. *Epilepsy: A Practical Guide to Coping*, Crowood Press, London, 1989.

Scambler, G. *Epilepsy*, Routledge, London, 1989.

Schacter, SC. *Brainstorms: Epilepsy in Our Words* [personal accounts of living with seizures], Raven Press, New York, 1993.

Whitman, S & Hermann BP. *Psychopathology in Epilepsy – Social Dimensions*, Oxford University Press, Oxford, 1986.

Yanko, S. *Coming to Terms with Epilepsy*, Allen & Unwin, Sydney, 1993.

Index

Absence seizures
  choice of drug, 32
  typical/atypical, 8–9
Acceptance
  by patient, 75–6
  by society, 76–9
  stigmatization of
    epileptic, 75–80
Aetiology of epilepsy,
    13–15
  by age, 14
Air travel, 83
Alcohol intake, 54
Anti-epileptic drugs, 28–55
  commencement, 28–9,
    33–5
  compliance, 51–2
  developing drugs, 94
  information for patients,
    86–8
  length of treatment,
    29–30
  people with disabilities,
    65–6
  pregnancy, 63–5
  side-effects, 32–3
  teratogenicity, 65
  therapeutic drug
    monitoring, 50
  withdrawal of treatment,
    30–1
  see also specific drugs
Australia

Epilepsy Associations,
    98–9
  epilepsy centres, 95–6

Bathing and showering,
    82
Behavioural disturbances,
    72–3
Benign familial neonatal
    seizures, prognosis,
    5
Benign focal epilepsy *see*
    Benign partial
    epilepsy with
    centrotemporal
    spikes
Benign neonatal seizures,
    prognosis and
    outcome, 5
Benign partial epilepsy
    with centrotemporal
    spikes, 9–10
Bicycling, 82
Blood tests, 27, 87
Breast feeding, 65

Carbamazepine
  characteristics and use,
    36
  in partial epilepsy, 10
  side-effects, 36

Childhood and juvenile syndromes
  characteristics, 5–12
  classification, 4
  management, 61–2
  seizure-free period, 30
  seizures in, 52
Classification, 1–12
  childhood and juvenile syndromes, 4
  ILAE, 2–4
Clobazam
  characteristics and use, 37
  side-effects, 37
Clonazepam
  characteristics and use, 38
  side-effects, 38
Cognitive problems, 74
  and pseudo-epileptic seizures, 68
Computerized tomography (CT) scanning, 21–4
Computers, 67
Concealment of epilepsy, 79–80
Cooking, 83
Corpus callosotomy, 57–8

Diagnosis, 18–27
  neurological examination, 19–26
Diazepam
  characteristics, 39
  side-effects, 39
Disabilities, 65–6
Driving, 84

Elderly patients, management, 62–3
Electroencephalography, 20–1
Emotional disorders, 73
Employment, 84–5
Epilepsy
  concealment, 79–80
  differentiation from pseudo-epileptic seizures, 69–70
  epidemiology, 15–16
  incidence, 15
  inheritance, 63–4
  lifestyle aspects, 81–8
  recurrence rates, 16–17
  seizure-free period, 30
  stigmatization of epileptic, 73, 75–80
Epilepsy Associations
  Australia, 98–9
  Ireland, 101
  New Zealand, 100–101
  UK, 101
Epilepsy centres, 95–7
Ethosuximide
  characteristics, 40
  side-effects, 40

Febrile convulsions
  defined, 8
  prognosis, 7–8
Felbamate
  characteristics and use, 41
  Lennox–Gastaut syndrome, 7
  side-effects, 41
  uncertainties, 32
Folic acid, 65

Index

Gabapentin
  characteristics and use, 42
  side-effects, 42
Generalized seizures
  choice of drug, 32
  classification, 1, 2–4
Generalized tonic–clonic seizures
  on awakening, 11–12, 32
  choice of drug, 32
Grief reaction, 76
GTCS *see* Generalized tonic–clonic seizures

Hemispherectomy, 58
Hidden distress model, 79
Horse-riding, 83

Infantile spasms *see* West syndrome
Information for patients, 86–8
Inheritance of epilepsy, 63–4
Ireland, Epilepsy Associations, 101

Juvenile myoclonic epilepsy
  characteristics, 10
  choice of drug, 32
  prognosis and outcome, 10–11

Lamotrigine
  characteristics and use, 43
  commencement, 33–4
  in Lennox–Gastaut syndrome, 7
  side-effects, 43
Lennox–Gastaut syndrome, prognosis, 7
Lifestyle aspects of epilepsy, 81–8
Light sensitivity, 54, 66–7

Magnetic resonance imaging (MRI), 21, 23, 25
Mesial temporal sclerosis, 8
Metabolic causes
  epilepsy, 15
  neonatal seizures, 61
Myoclonic epilepsy in infancy, benign/severe, prognosis and outcome, 6

Neonatal seizures
  causes
    first–fourth days, 60
    metabolic causes, 61
  classification, 4, 60
  status epilepticus, 52
Neuro-imaging, indications, 21
Neurological examination, 19–26
Neurotube defects, 65
New Zealand, Epilepsy Associations, 100–101
Non-compliance, 51–2

Occupational hazards, 84–5
Oxcarbazepine
  characteristics and use, 44
  side-effects, 44

Paroxysmal depolarization shift (PDS), defined, 13
Partial seizures
  with centrotemporal spikes, 9–10
  choice of drug, 32
  complex (CPS)
    classification, 1, 2
    CT and MRI guidelines, 23–6
  simple (SPS)
    classification, 1, 2
    CT scanning guidelines, 22
Phenobarbitone, characteristics and side-effects, 45
Phenytoin, characteristics and side-effects, 46
Photosensitivity, 54, 66–7
Piracetam, 94
Positron emission tomography (PET), 21
Pregnancy, effects of epilepsy, 63–5
Primidone, characteristics and side-effects, 47
Prognosis of epilepsy, 15–17
Pseudo-epileptic seizures, 68–71
  compared with epilepsy, 69–70
  diagnosis, 71
  and intellect, 68
  precipitating causes, 69
Psychosocial issues, 72–80
Pyridoxine dependency, prognosis and outcome, 5–6

Recurrence rates, 16–17
References, 89–93
  further reading, 102
Remacimide, 94

Schools, epilepsy centres, 97
Seizure-free period
  adults, 30
  children, 30
Seizures
  behavioural disturbances, 72–3
  classification, 1–12
  defined, 1
  emotional disorders, 73
Sexual abuse, 71
Sexuality, 74
Single photon emission computed tomography (SPECT), 21
Sleep
  advice, 83
  generalized tonic–clonic seizures on awakening, 11–12, 32
Sleep deprivation, 54